Steatosis - Causes and Treatment

Edited by Costin Teodor Streba

Published in London, United Kingdom

Steatosis - Causes and Treatment
http://dx.doi.org/10.5772/intechopen.1007990
Edited by Costin Teodor Streba

Contributors
Aamir Sohail, Adina-Dorina Glodeanu, Aleena Altaf, Alexandre S. Rosado, Alexandru Sidencu, Anca Mihu-Marinescu, Basak Celtikci, Borna AliBabazadeh, Chang Liu, Consolato M. Sergi, Cristina Florescu, Diana-Maria Trașcă, Diana-Ruxandra Hădăreanu, Edme-Roxana Mustafa, Elena Gologan, Faisal M. Sanai, Faiza Noreen, Fatemeh Maleki Sedgi, Hamza Muneer, Huiling Gao, Idrees Raza, Imran Ullah, Ion-Cristian Efrem, Iulian-Alin-Silviu Popescu, Lilia Lica, Linah Aljahdali, Maimoona Arshad, Mete Ucdal, Muhammad Asim, Muhammad Murtaza Hasnain, Mutep Aljahdali, Oana Timofte, Raza Sufyan, Rodica Pădureanu, Shan Gao, Sorina Ionelia Stan, Veronica Gheorman, Viorel Biciușcă, Vlad Pădureanu, Wesam Bahitham, Yaoxin Wu, Yusra Banoun

First published in London, United Kingdom, 2025 by IntechOpen
IntechOpen is the global imprint of INTECHOPEN LIMITED, registered in England and Wales, registration number: 11086078, 167-169 Great Portland Street, London, W1W 5PF, United Kingdom

For EU product safety concerns: IN TECH d.o.o., Prolaz Marije Krucifikse Kozulić 3, 51000 Rijeka, Croatia, info@intechopen.com or visit our website at intechopen.com.

British Library Cataloguing-in-Publication Data
A catalogue record for this book is available from the British Library

Steatosis - Causes and Treatment
Edited by Costin Teodor Streba
p. cm.
Print ISBN 978-1-83635-355-3
Online ISBN 978-1-83635-354-6
eBook (PDF) ISBN 978-1-83635-356-0

If disposing of this product, please recycle the paper responsibly.

Meet the editor

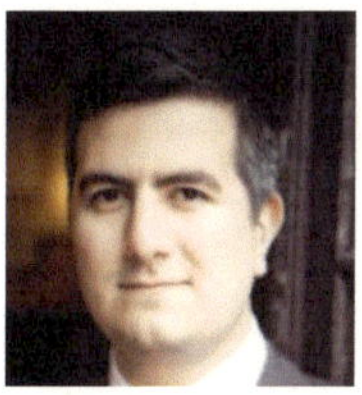

Costin Teodor Streba, MD, Ph.D., MSc, is a professor at the University of Medicine and Pharmacy of Craiova, Romania, and a member of the university's Research Center of Gastroenterology and Hepatology of Craiova. He has extensive research experience in the diagnosis and treatment of liver and pancreatic diseases, as well as training in histological image analysis. He specialized in devising medical-oriented diagnostic systems for liver malignancies that integrate interpretation and computer-aided quantification of various imaging and clinical data. Dr. Teodor has published extensively on innovative diagnostic techniques in gastroenterology.

Contents

Preface

This Edited Volume is a collection of reviewed and relevant research chapters concerning the developments within the field of study of steatosis. The book features scholarly contributions from various authors and is edited by an expert in the field. Each contribution comes as a separate chapter complete in itself but directly related to the book's topics and objectives.

The book is divided into two sections: *From Bench to Bedside – Integrative Overview of MAFLD and Lifestyle* and *Medical Intervention in MAFLD*.

The target audience comprises scholars and specialists in the field.

IntechOpen

Section 1

From Bench to Bedside – Integrative Overview of MAFLD

Chapter 1

Perspective Chapter: Cross-Talk between Genetics and Biochemistry in the Pathogenesis of Hepatic Steatosis

Mete Ucdal and Basak Celtikci

Abstract

Hepatic steatosis development involves intricate interactions between genetic susceptibility and biochemical pathway dysregulation. This chapter examines the molecular foundations of hepatocellular lipid accumulation, focusing on metabolic networks and cell death mechanisms. Genetic polymorphisms in lipid regulatory genes (PNPLA3, TM6SF2, and MBOAT7) significantly influence metabolic enzyme expression patterns. Central biochemical processes examined include de novo lipogenesis, β-oxidation impairment, and triglyceride export dysfunction. Particular emphasis is placed on ferrinophagy—a specialized autophagic process regulating iron homeostasis—and its relationship to oxidative stress in steatotic hepatocytes. Further analysis explores how metabolic death pathways, including pyroptosis and necroptosis, contribute to disease progression and potential therapeutic targeting opportunities.

Keywords: hepatic steatosis, genetic predisposition, metabolic pathways, ferrinophagycell death mechanisms, metabolomics, transcriptomics

1. Introduction

Non-alcoholic fatty liver disease (NAFLD), recently redefined as metabolic dysfunction-associated fatty liver disease (MAFLD), has become the most common chronic liver condition worldwide, affecting roughly a quarter of the adult population [1]. MAFLD encompasses a spectrum from simple steatosis (fatty liver) to metabolic dysfunction-associated steatohepatitis (MASH) and fibrosis and can progress to cirrhosis and hepatocellular carcinoma (HCC) [2]. It is tightly associated with metabolic comorbidities including obesity, type 2 diabetes mellitus (T2DM), dyslipidemia, and insulin resistance [3]. Indeed, up to 80–90% of obese individuals and ~ 60% of those with T2DM have evidence of NAFLD, underscoring that metabolic dysfunction is a key driver of hepatic steatosis [4]. Genetic predispositions (e.g., variants in *PNPLA3*, *TM6SF2*, *HSD17B13*, and others) modify individual susceptibility, but the pathogenesis is largely orchestrated by metabolic and biochemical disturbances [5].

These metabolic derangements—excess caloric intake, altered carbohydrate and lipid handling, amino acid imbalances, iron overload, and mitochondrial dysfunction—create a lipotoxic and pro-inflammatory hepatic milieu that triggers cell injury and death pathways [6].

Hepatocyte death is now recognized as a critical turning point that drives the transition from benign steatosis to inflammation (NASH) and fibrosis in MAFLD [7]. Traditionally, hepatocyte apoptosis (programmed cell death mediated by caspases -3/-7 *via* death receptors or ER stress) was viewed as the predominant mode of cell death in NASH [8]. However, over the past decade, research has revealed that other forms of regulated cell death (RCD)—notably pyroptosis, necroptosis, and ferroptosis—play major roles in the progression of fatty liver disease [9]. *Pyroptosis* is an inflammatory form of cell death triggered by inflammasome activation and caspase-1, leading to gasdermin pore formation, cell lysis, and release of IL-1β and IL-18 [10]. *Necroptosis* is a caspase-independent, TNF-mediated cell death pathway involving receptor-interacting protein kinases (RIPK1/RIPK3) and MLKL, resulting in membrane rupture and release of damage-associated molecular patterns (DAMPs) [11]. *Ferroptosis* is a distinct iron-dependent cell death caused by overwhelming lipid peroxidation and reactive oxygen species (ROS) accumulation when antioxidant defenses (like glutathione peroxidase 4, GPX4) fail [12]. These death pathways are inherently linked to metabolic stress: for example, nutrient excess and lipotoxicity activate inflammasomes (pyroptosis) and death receptors (necroptosis), while iron overload and glutathione depletion precipitate ferroptosis [13]. Importantly, pyroptosis and necroptosis are lytic, pro-inflammatory cell deaths that amplify liver inflammation, and ferroptosis induces massive oxidative injury; all three can trigger fibrogenic responses in the liver [14].

Apoptosis is a form of programmed cell death executed by caspases. In hepatocytes, extrinsic apoptosis is typically initiated by death ligands (TNF-α, FasL, TRAIL) binding to their receptors (TNFR, Fas, and TRAIL-R) and recruiting adaptor proteins to form the death-inducing signaling complex (DISC), leading to activation of caspase-8 and downstream effector caspases-3/-7. Intrinsic apoptosis can be triggered by metabolic stress (e.g., ER stress and oxidative stress), causing mitochondrial outer membrane permeabilization (MOMP) and cytochrome c release, which activates caspase-9 and then caspase-3/-7. Both pathways result in DNA fragmentation and cell death without cell lysis, in contrast to the inflammatory cell lysis seen in pyroptosis and necroptosis. Apoptosis has been widely observed in NASH, but recent evidence highlights that non-apoptotic cell death pathways (pyroptosis, necroptosis, ferroptosis) also contribute significantly to disease progression [8, 11].

An emerging concept is that hepatocytes in NASH may undergo multiple RCD pathways simultaneously or sequentially in response to chronic metabolic insults. In some contexts, the three inflammatory RCD modalities (pyroptosis, necroptosis, and apoptosis) can co-occur, a phenomenon termed *Panoptosis*, involving cross-talk among their signaling mechanisms [15]. This chapter explores the cross-talk between metabolic dysfunction and regulated cell death in the pathogenesis of hepatic steatosis. We structure the discussion around five key metabolic axes—carbohydrate metabolism, lipid metabolism, protein/amino acid metabolism, iron metabolism, and mitochondrial function—to illustrate how perturbations in each axis trigger and amplify pyroptosis, necroptosis, and ferroptosis in hepatocytes. We also highlight how these processes, in concert with metabolic comorbidities, drive progression from simple steatosis to NASH, fibrosis, and HCC. Mechanistic insights from the last 5–10 years are emphasized, and clinical correlations are drawn to common metabolic disorders (obesity,

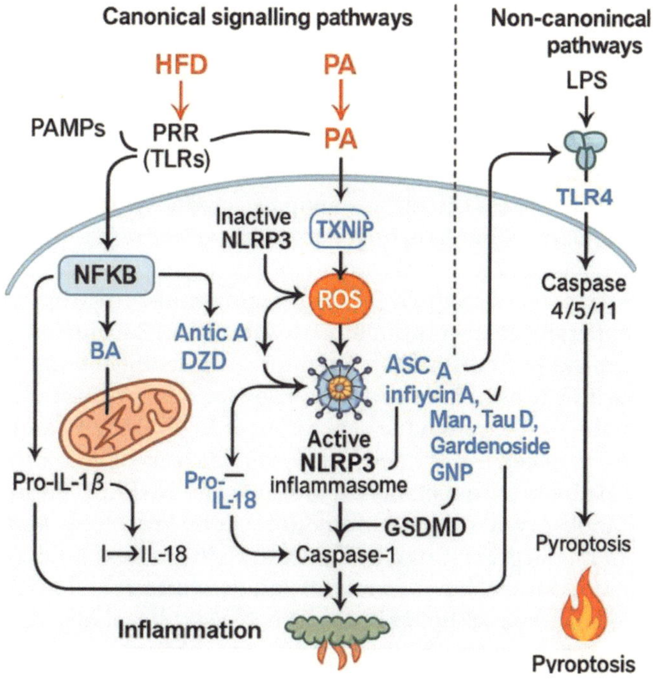

Figure 1.
Mechanisms of hepatocyte apoptosis in NAFLD.

T2DM, dyslipidemia), underscoring the translational relevance of these cell death pathways in MAFLD. Figures are provided to map metabolism–cell death relationships (e.g., "metabolic checkpoints in hepatocyte pyroptosis"), and summary tables compile key molecular players and potential therapeutic interventions (**Figure 1**).

2. Carbohydrate metabolism and hepatocyte injury in MAFLD

Overconsumption of simple carbohydrates, particularly fructose-rich foods, and sugar-sweetened beverages, is strongly linked to the development of fatty liver and NASH. Excess dietary carbohydrates drive hyperinsulinemia and insulin resistance, which in turn dysregulate glucose and lipid homeostasis. The liver, as a central hub of carbohydrate metabolism, is directly impacted by chronic glycemic and insulin perturbations. Two major consequences of carbohydrate overload in MAFLD are heightened de novo lipogenesis (conversion of carbs to fatty acids) and a state of chronic mild inflammation often referred to as metabolic endotoxemia [16]. These consequences create a pro-death environment in the liver by supplying lipotoxic substrates and inflammatory stimuli that can trigger hepatocyte death programs.

Insulin resistance and excess glucose: In the insulin-resistant state of obesity and T2DM, hepatocytes are bombarded with both glucose and free fatty acids (due to uninhibited adipose lipolysis). High intracellular glucose can disturb cellular redox balance and carbon fluxes. Enhanced glycolysis and tricarboxylic acid (TCA) cycle activity lead to mitochondrial overload and increased ROS generation [17]. Hyperglycemia also promotes the formation of advanced glycation end-products (AGEs) and activation of the receptor for AGE (RAGE), eliciting inflammatory signaling in hepatocytes and Kupffer cells [18]. Oxidative stress from glucose excess can damage mitochondria and release mitochondrial DNA (mtDNA) and other DAMPs into the cytosol, which are potent triggers of the inflammasome and cell death pathways (discussed below) [19]. In parallel, chronic hyperinsulinemia suppresses autophagy and promotes ER stress in hepatocytes by driving protein and lipid synthesis; these conditions sensitize cells to injury. The unfolded protein response (UPR) triggered by ER stress can initiate apoptotic pathways *via* CHOP, but it also intersects with inflammasome signaling. For instance, excess glucose and insulin signaling increase hepatic TXNIP (thioredoxin-interacting protein), an intracellular sensor that links oxidative stress to NLRP3 inflammasome activation [20]. TXNIP is upregulated in hyperglycemia and can directly bind NLRP3, contributing to its activation and subsequent pyroptosis [20]. Therefore, the derangements of carbohydrate metabolism in insulin-resistant states set the stage for both apoptotic and inflammatory cell death in the liver through the generation of ROS, DAMPs, and stress signals. Clinically, this is evidenced by elevated circulating markers of oxidative stress and inflammation in patients with metabolic syndrome and NAFLD (**Figure 2**) [21].

Fructose metabolism and inflammasome activation: Fructose is a particularly lipogenic sugar that is largely cleared by the liver. High fructose intake (e.g., from sweetened drinks) has been shown to rapidly induce steatosis and inflammation in experimental models, even without obesity. Fructose is phosphorylated by ketohexokinase in hepatocytes, depleting ATP and generating AMP that is metabolized to uric acid. The resultant uric acid and ATP depletion are themselves danger signals that can activate inflammasomes in the liver [22]. Uric acid crystals and excess intracellular AMP can trigger the NOD-like receptor protein 3 (NLRP3) inflammasome in macrophages/Kupffer cells, leading to caspase-1 activation and maturation of IL-1β and IL-18 cytokines (hallmarks of pyroptosis) [22]. Fructose metabolism also causes oxidative stress and gut dysbiosis: it increases gut permeability and enables endotoxin

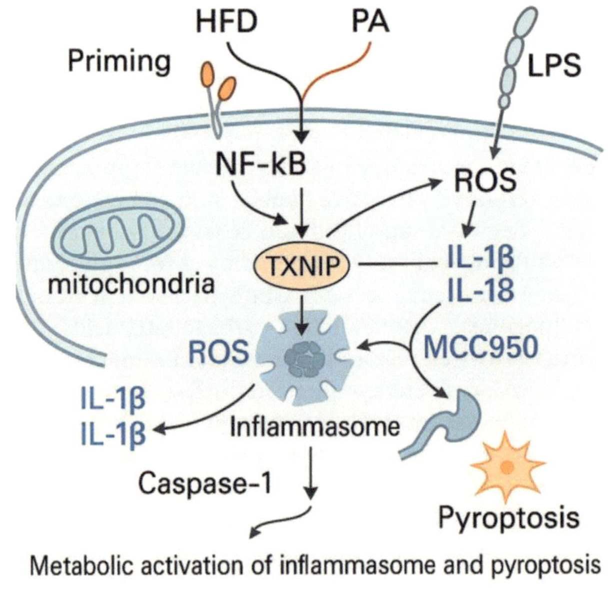

Figure 2.
Metabolic activation of the inflammasome and pyroptosis in NAFLD.

(LPS) translocation from the intestine to the liver *via* the portal circulation. Even in the absence of infection, a high-fructose or high-fat diet can elevate portal LPS levels (so-called metabolic endotoxemia), which engages Toll-like receptor-4 (TLR4) on Kupffer cells, providing a potent priming signal for inflammasome assembly [23]. Together, these effects mean that fructose can drive sterile inflammation in the liver akin to an innate immune response. Studies in mice have demonstrated that fructose feeding leads to the upregulation of inflammasome components (NLRP3, ASC, and caspase-1) and increased hepatic IL-1β and that this is associated with hepatocyte pyroptotic cell death and worsening liver injury [24]. Inhibiting NLRP3 activation (genetically or with small-molecule inhibitors like MCC950) has been shown to alleviate fructose-induced steatohepatitis, confirming that the inflammasome–pyroptosis pathway mediates much of the damage [24]. Clinically, patients with MAFLD who consume high fructose diets have been found to have higher levels of inflammasome-related cytokines and a more inflammatory MASH phenotype [25].

3. Lipid metabolism and lipotoxicity-driven cell death in fatty liver disease

Disturbances in carbohydrate metabolism—notably insulin resistance and high fructose/glucose exposure—promote hepatocyte injury largely by supplying excess substrates that drive *lipogenesis, oxidative stress, and inflammation*, which converge on the *inflammasome–pyroptosis pathway*. While pyroptotic activity is prominent, apoptosis and necroptosis also occur in this setting: for instance, prolonged ER stress from nutrient excess can lead to hepatocyte apoptosis, and extreme ATP depletion (as can happen with fructose overdose) may cause necrotic cell death. However, it is the *inflammatory death* component that distinguishes carbohydrate-driven liver injury. Clinically, this is why patients with poorly controlled diabetes or high-sugar diets often exhibit elevated liver inflammation markers and progress more rapidly to MASH [3, 25, 26]. Controlling carbohydrate intake and improving insulin sensitivity (e.g., *via* diet, metformin, and GLP-1 agonists) have been shown to lower hepatic IL-1β levels and histological NASH activity in trials, which is consistent with dampening the pyroptosis-inflammasome axis by reversing the upstream metabolic triggers [27]. Carbohydrate metabolism thus sets the stage for liver cell death by creating an environment rich in inflammatory triggers, making it a fundamental axis in MAFLD pathogenesis.

Excessive lipid accumulation in the liver is the hallmark of MAFLD, and dysregulated lipid metabolism is central to hepatocellular injury. In the context of obesity and overnutrition, the liver is flooded with fatty acids from dietary fat, adipose tissue lipolysis (enhanced by insulin resistance), and de novo lipogenesis. While some fatty acids are stored benignly as triglycerides within lipid droplets, a significant proportion give rise to lipotoxic species—free fatty acids (especially saturated fats), free cholesterol, and other lipid metabolites (diacylglycerols and ceramides)—that can disrupt cellular membranes and organelles [29]. Lipotoxic stress directly triggers hepatocyte death pathways: saturated fatty acids can induce ER stress and mitochondrial dysfunction, cholesterol can activate immune pathways in Kupffer cells, and oxidized lipids generate ROS. Three major death modalities are linked to lipid toxicity in NAFLD: apoptosis (sometimes termed lipoapoptosis in this setting), necroptosis, and ferroptosis. Additionally, lipids can indirectly provoke pyroptosis *via* inflammation. In this section, we examine how derangements in lipid metabolism—from fatty acid overload to impaired lipid export—lead to these forms of cell death.

Saturated versus unsaturated fatty acids (FFA): Hepatocytes exposed to high levels of FFAs undergo profound stress. Saturated FFA (such as palmitate and abundant in high-fat diets) are especially toxic: they are known to insert into the plasma and organelle membranes, causing membrane saturation and rigidity, which perturbs the function of the ER and mitochondria [30]. Palmitate triggers the unfolded protein response in the ER; if this stress is severe or prolonged, it activates apoptosis *via* CHOP and JNK signaling. Simultaneously, saturated FFA overloading of mitochondria leads to incomplete β-oxidation and excess electron leakage, producing ROS that can damage mitochondrial DNA and proteins [31]. These conditions favor cell death over adaptation.

By contrast, monounsaturated FFA (like oleate) are better tolerated because they can be more readily esterified into triglycerides for storage or export, and they can actually attenuate palmitate toxicity by promoting safe lipid droplet formation [29]. This dichotomy is evident *in vitro*: hepatocytes incubated with palmitate show high rates of apoptosis and membrane rupture, whereas co-supplementation with oleate reduces cell death [30]. Thus, the quality of fatty acids impact which death pathways are engaged—saturated fats tilt toward apoptosis/necroptosis, whereas unsaturated fats channel into neutral lipid storage and less cell death. In obesity, diets often contain excess saturated fats, contributing to the lipotoxic burden on the liver and priming cell death mechanisms.

Lipotoxic activation of death receptors and necroptosis: A remarkable feature of lipotoxic stress in metabolic dysfunction-associated steatohepatitis (MASH) is its ability to activate death receptor pathways, particularly the TNF pathway. Hepatocytes overloaded with lipotoxic species often upregulates death receptors like Fas and secrete TNFα from stressed cells or neighboring Kupffer cells [32]. Upon exposure to lipotoxic stress (e.g., palmitic acid or choline-deficient diets leading to steatosis), these cells produce death ligands that bind to their cognate receptors.

The binding of TNF-α to TNFR1, or FasL to Fas, initiates the formation of Complex I (containing TRADD, TRAF2/5, RIPK1, and other adaptors). In metabolically healthy cells, this either activates NF-κB signaling for survival or, if it forms Complex II, leads to caspase-8 activation and controlled apoptosis. However, in MASH, multiple factors disrupt this normal signaling cascade. Oxidative stress (ROS, elevated in fatty liver), ER stress (e.g., ATF3 induction by saturated fat), and lipotoxicity itself can inhibit caspase-8 activity, creating what is known as a "Complex IIb scenario" [11].

This caspase-8 inhibition (which can also result from pharmacologic inhibitors or FADD absence) allows RIPK1 and RIPK3 to interact and phosphorylate each other, assembling the necrosome complex. Studies have found that in fatty livers, caspase-8 activity is paradoxically lowered despite strong TNF signaling, thereby shunting cells toward necroptosis rather than apoptosis [33]. RIPK3 then phosphorylates MLKL (mixed lineage kinase domain-like protein), which oligomerizes and translocates to the plasma membrane, forming pores that lead to cell swelling and rupture. This necroptotic cell death releases intracellular contents including damage-associated molecular patterns (DAMPs like HMGB1, mitochondrial DNA) that amplify inflammation [11].

Several metabolic factors specifically promote necroptosis in MAFLD. Palmitate (PA) and the transcription factor ATF3 upregulate RIPK3; methionine-choline deficient (MCD) diets and intermittent hypoxia (IH, mimicking obstructive sleep apnea) both increase hepatic RIPK3 and MLKL activation in NASH models, aggravating liver injury [35, 36]. Additionally, saturated FFA can activate JNK, which has been shown to promote necroptosis by upregulating death receptors and potentially interfering with caspase-8 function [34]. TLR4 activation by LPS (common in obesity-associated endotoxemia) can also feed into RIPK3 activation *via* TRIF, providing another route for necroptosis induction.

Therapeutic approaches targeting this pathway include RIPK1 inhibitors like RIPA-56, RIPK3 inhibitors such as GSK-872, and dual PPAR agonists like elafibranor (ELA), which have shown hepatoprotective effects by reducing necroptosis in preclinical studies [33, 35]. The culmination of necroptosis—membrane rupture and release of DAMPs—drives inflammation, creating a feed-forward cycle of injury that distinguishes it from the "cleaner" apoptotic death. This mechanism illustrates how metabolic stress (steatosis, ROS) redirects TNF signaling away from apoptosis toward necroptosis in fatty livers (**Figure 3**).

In a high-fat-fed mouse model, genetic deletion of RIPK3 or MLKL significantly reduced liver injury and inflammation, indicating that necroptosis contributes to hepatocyte death in MASH [35]. Correspondingly, human MASH livers exhibit increased RIPK3 and MLKL expression compared to simple steatosis or healthy livers, and these correlate with disease severity [35]. Necroptosis is particularly relevant to the transition from steatosis to steatohepatitis—when hepatocyte fat content is high, a toxic stimulus like excess TNF or LPS can trigger widespread necroptotic death, releasing DAMPs that incite inflammation. This helps explain the clinical observation that MAFLD patients with higher circulating TNF levels or adipocytokines often have worse liver injury.

In addition to fatty acids, free cholesterol accumulation in the liver has deleterious effects. Cholesterol is normally exported in lipoproteins or converted to bile acids,

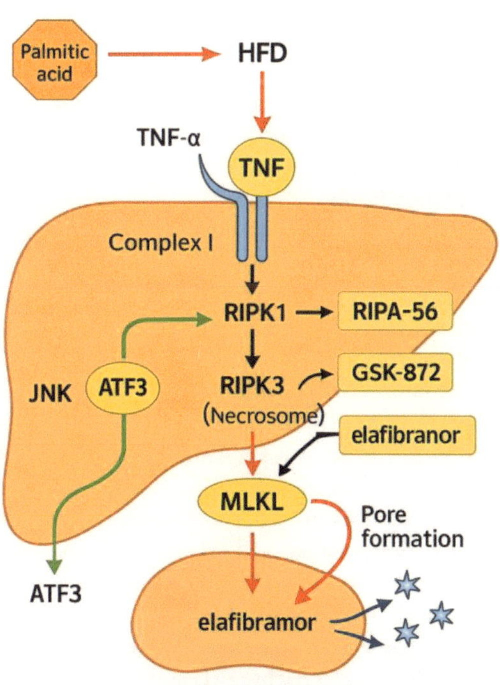

Figure 3.
Mechanism of hepatocyte necroptosis under lipotoxic and inflammatory conditions.

but in Metabolic dysfunction-Associated SteatoHepatitis (MASH) these pathways can be impaired, leading to cholesterol deposition in hepatocytes and Kupffer cells. Excess free cholesterol in hepatocyte membranes stiffens the membranes and can induce a form of stress that triggers apoptosis *via* mitochondrial cholesterol loading and permeability transition [37]. More prominently, cholesterol crystals can form in Kupffer cells and activate the NLRP3 inflammasome, similar to processes observed in atherosclerotic plaque macrophages [24]. Kupffer cells overloaded with cholesterol become a source of IL-1β *via* inflammasome activation, which can induce pyroptosis in those macrophages and amplify inflammatory signaling to hepatocytes and stellate cells [24]. Thus, dysregulated cholesterol metabolism provides another link between lipids and the pyroptosis pathway. In human MASH, studies have found crystallized cholesterol deposits in liver tissue that correlate with lobular inflammation and fibrosis, supporting the concept that cholesterol-driven inflammasome activation contributes to disease severity [38].

One aspect of lipid metabolism in MAFLD is the ability of the liver to export triglycerides as VLDL. When this capacity is exceeded due to overwhelming lipid influx or deficiencies in export factors like choline, hepatocytes accumulate fat and become vulnerable to lipoapoptosis—apoptosis due to fat-induced cell stress. Key mediators of lipoapoptosis are the JNK pathway and the Bcl-2 family proteins. Saturated free fatty acids can activate JNK, which then phosphorylates and inactivates insulin receptor substrates (worsening insulin resistance) but also phosphorylates pro-apoptotic proteins like BIM, tipping the balance toward apoptosis [34].

n steatotic hepatocytes, JNK activation and upregulation of pro-apoptotic Bax and PUMA have been observed alongside increases in caspase-3 activity, indicating apoptosis in action [30]. Lipoapoptosis specifically describes how fat triggers the intrinsic mitochondrial pathway: excess fatty acids cause Bax/Bak insertion into the mitochondria, cytochrome c release, and caspase-3 activation, leading to DNA fragmentation and cell death [37]. Evidence for lipoapoptosis in patients comes from biopsies showing TUNEL-positive cells in zones of high steatosis and from elevated serum cytokeratin-18 fragments (a marker of hepatocyte apoptosis) in MASH patients compared to simple steatosis [39]. While apoptosis is a "silent" cell death, in a fatty liver, it is not entirely benign—apoptotic bodies from hepatocytes can be engulfed by stellate cells and Kupffer cells, which then become activated and produce collagen and cytokines, linking to fibrosis and inflammation [8].

Necroptosis has emerged as a major contributor to lipotoxic liver injury. Mice fed a high-fat, choline-deficient diet for 18 weeks had marked increases in MLKL and RIPK3 activation in their livers and developed more severe steatohepatitis compared to wild-type controls; however, in MLKL-knockout mice, the same diet resulted in significantly less liver inflammation and injury [35]. This indicates necroptotic hepatocyte death was driving much of the injury. Another study reported that hepatocyte-specific deletion of RIPK3 protected mice from high-fat diet MASH and also reduced fibrosis, suggesting that necroptosis of hepatocytes is a fibrogenic stimulus, likely through the DAMPs and cytokines released [33].

In humans, clinical studies found hepatic RIPK3 mRNA levels were higher in patients with MASH than in those with simple fatty liver, and higher in those with fibrosis than those without, consistent with animal data [35]. These findings collectively position necroptosis as a key pathway by which lipid overload translates into cell death and inflammation. Conditions that commonly accompany obesity can exacerbate necroptosis. Intermittent hypoxia (as occurs in obstructive sleep apnea, prevalent in obese individuals) was found to aggravate MAFLD *via* RIPK3-dependent necroptosis—chronic intermittent hypoxia increased RIPK3/MLKL activation in the liver, leading to more cell death and MASH progression in mice [36].

Therapies targeting the TNF-RIPK3-MLKL axis are being explored; for example, Necrostatin-1 (a RIPK1 inhibitor) and RIPK3 inhibitors have shown a reduction of liver injury in MASH models [33]. Some existing drugs have anti-necroptotic effects: the dual PPARα/δ agonist elafibranor appears to reduce necroptosis by modulating RIPK signaling, and omega-3 fatty acids or PPAR agonists can reduce JNK activation and may indirectly mitigate necroptosis [34, 35].

Lipid overload inherently leads to oxidative stress—excess β-oxidation in mitochondria and peroxisomes generates H_2O_2, and cytochrome P450 oxidation of fatty acids in microsomes generates free radicals. When antioxidant systems are overwhelmed, highly reactive lipid peroxides accumulate. This can initiate ferroptosis, especially if iron is abundant. In steatotic hepatocytes, studies have noted reduced expression of GPX4 and depleted glutathione levels, rendering cells susceptible to iron-catalyzed lipid peroxidation [40].

Certain lipid metabolic changes in MASH favor ferroptosis; for instance, an increase in polyunsaturated fatty acids in hepatocyte membranes provides an abundant substrate for peroxidation. Livers of MASH patients often contain elevated levels of lipid peroxidation markers (malondialdehyde and 4-hydroxynonenal), indicating ongoing lipid peroxidation damage [41]. Over 90% of MAFLD patients have higher-than-normal hepatic MDA and 4-HNE levels, and those with MASH have significantly more than those with simple steatosis [41].

Recent studies implicate ferroptosis in MASH: in a methionine-choline deficient diet model, treating mice with the ferroptosis inhibitor liproxstatin-1 or an iron chelator (deferoxamine) markedly reduced liver injury, inflammation, and fibrosis, whereas inducing ferroptosis (with RSL3, a GPX4 inhibitor) worsened MASH severity [42]. This provides strong evidence that lipid peroxidation-driven death is occurring in fatty livers and is not merely a byproduct of damage.

The death of hepatocytes due to lipotoxicity does not happen in isolation; it triggers an inflammatory response that further perturbs lipid metabolism. Necroptotic hepatocytes release HMGB1, which can bind TLR4 on Kupffer cells, causing them to produce more TNFα and IL-1β, feeding a cycle of ongoing cell death and inflammation [11, 33]. Similarly, if hepatocytes undergo ferroptosis, the released lipid peroxidation products can activate stellate cells and Kupffer cells, inducing them to secrete pro-inflammatory and pro-fibrotic mediators. Thus, the initial metabolic insult leads to cell death, which then exacerbates metabolic dysfunction in the liver *via* inflammation. This is one reason MASH can become self-sustaining even if the original metabolic trigger plateaus—the damaged liver environment itself perpetuates further injury.

Dysregulated lipid metabolism in MAFLD (characterized by free fatty acid overload, cholesterol accumulation, and impaired lipid export) is a principal instigator of hepatocyte death. Lipotoxicity inflicts cellular stress that activates intrinsic apoptosis, necroptosis *via* death receptor signals, and ferroptosis *via* oxidative damage. Each of these death pathways has been demonstrated in experimental MASH and correlated with human disease severity. The net result of lipid-driven cell death is the transition of a fatty but relatively quiescent liver into an inflamed, injured organ (steatohepatitis).

Clinically, patients with elevated free fatty acid levels or those with high dietary saturated fat intake tend to have more aggressive MASH, highlighting the connection between lipid metabolism and liver cell death [3, 29]. Therapeutically, interventions that reduce hepatic lipotoxicity (weight loss, dietary modification to reduce saturated

Metabolic perturbation	Affected cell death pathway	Mechanistic effect and outcome
Chronic hyperglycemia, insulin resistance	Pyroptosis (inflammasome activation); apoptosis	↑ROS and DAMPs trigger NLRP3 inflammasome → IL-1β release and pyroptotic inflammation; ER stress (*via* CHOP) induces apoptotic cascades [17, 20]
High fructose intake, gut endotoxemia	Pyroptosis (inflammasome activation)	Fructose metabolism depletes ATP, ↑uric acid and gut LPS → activates Kupffer cell NLRP3 → caspase-1/GSDMD-mediated hepatocyte pyroptosis and cytokine release [22, 24]
Saturated fatty acid excess (lipotoxicity)	Apoptosis; necroptosis; pyroptosis	Palmitate causes ER stress and JNK activation → mitochondrial apoptosis; also ↑TNF/JNK → caspase-8 inhibition → RIPK3/MLKL necroptosis; palmitate/TLR4 → priming of inflammasome (pyroptosis) [30, 33]
Free cholesterol accumulation	Apoptosis; pyroptosis (*via* inflammasome)	Mitochondrial cholesterol induces membrane permeability → apoptosis; cholesterol crystals in Kupffer cells activate NLRP3 → IL-1β release and secondary hepatocyte pyroptosis [24, 37]
Methionine/choline deficiency (impaired VLDL export)	Apoptosis; ferroptosis; necroptosis	Severe steatosis with depleted glutathione (methionine is GSH precursor) → vulnerable to lipid peroxidation and ferroptosis; ATP depletion and JNK activation in choline deficiency → necroptosis and apoptosis (as in MCD diet MASH) [34, 42]
Iron overload (high hepatic iron and ferritin)	Ferroptosis; amplifies others	Excess Fe^{2+} *via* Fenton reaction → massive lipid ROS → ferroptotic cell death; iron-driven ROS also serve as DAMPs to potentiate NLRP3 activation (pyroptosis) and sensitizes cells to TNF-induced necroptosis [40, 41]
Mitochondrial dysfunction (e.g., from obesity or hypoxia)	Apoptosis, necroptosis, and ferroptosis	Impaired β-oxidation → lipid accumulation and ROS → peroxidation (ferroptosis); mtDNA release and low ATP → NLRP3 activation (pyroptosis) and inability to execute apoptosis, favoring necroptosis; severe dysfunction causes MPT pore opening → necrosis [19, 36]

Table 1.
Metabolic perturbations and their effects on hepatocyte cell death pathways in MAFLD.

fat, or drugs that improve fat handling like PPAR agonists) have been shown to decrease hepatocyte apoptosis and necrosis in MASH biopsies, reinforcing the concept that mitigating metabolic lipid stress can prevent cell death and thereby slow disease progression (**Table 1**) [34, 39].

4. Protein and amino acid metabolism in MAFLD: Links to cell death

While much of the focus in MAFLD pathogenesis is on fats and sugars, disturbances in protein and amino acid metabolism also play a role in liver injury. The liver is central to amino acid catabolism (urea cycle and transamination), protein synthesis, and turnover (*via* autophagy and proteasomal degradation). In MAFLD, these processes can be altered by both nutrient excess and deficiency. Two aspects are particularly relevant: (1) deficiencies in specific nutrients (like choline and methionine) that impair hepatic lipid export and antioxidant capacity and (2) hyperaminoacidemia (elevated levels of certain amino acids) observed in insulin-resistant states that may exacerbate metabolic stress. Moreover, ER stress from protein misfolding and impaired autophagy (accumulation of protein aggregates and damaged organelles) are often found in MASH livers, linking protein metabolism to cell death. This section will discuss how these factors can trigger apoptosis, pyroptosis, and ferroptosis in the fatty liver.

Methionine and choline are essential nutrients crucial for hepatic lipid and one-carbon metabolism. Methionine is a precursor for S-adenosylmethionine (needed for phosphatidylcholine synthesis and DNA methylation) and for cysteine *via* the transsulfuration pathway (thus critical for glutathione production). Choline is required for synthesizing phosphatidylcholine, a component of VLDL particles that export triglycerides from the liver. Deficiency of either leads to impaired VLDL secretion and severe fat accumulation in hepatocytes.

The experimental methionine- and choline-deficient (MCD) diet is a well-established model of steatohepatitis characterized by marked steatosis, inflammation, and fibrosis. In this model, there is significant hepatocyte cell death driven by both apoptosis and ferroptosis. Methionine deficiency causes depletion of glutathione (because cysteine availability drops), leaving hepatocytes defenseless against oxidative injury [42]. Consequently, lipid peroxides accumulate unchecked, triggering ferroptosis. Indeed, treating MCD-fed mice with the ferroptosis inhibitor liproxstatin-1 or supplementing antioxidant selenium (to boost GPX4 activity) dramatically reduced liver damage, underscoring ferroptosis as a key death mechanism when methionine is lacking [42].

Choline deficiency, on the other hand, leads to massive triglyceride accumulation (because the liver cannot form VLDL without phosphatidylcholine). This extreme steatosis can cause mitochondrial dysfunction and cell lysis. It was shown that in a choline-deficient ethionine-supplemented (CDE) diet model, hepatocyte death occurred primarily through ferroptosis: inhibition of ferroptosis almost completely abrogated cell death, whereas necroptosis inhibition did not prevent it, suggesting ferroptosis was the initial mode of cell death in that scenario [43]. The CDE model is an aggressive fibrosing steatohepatitis model; Tsurusaki et al. found that ferroptosis inhibitors (but not necroptosis inhibitors) rescued hepatocytes from death, highlighting how a metabolic insult (choline deficiency with ethionine, which further disrupts methyl metabolism) engages ferroptosis early [43].

These findings imply that any condition that compromises glutathione or antioxidant systems (like deficiencies in methionine, cysteine, vitamin E, or selenium) can predispose the fatty liver to ferroptotic death. In patients, this might be relevant in cases of malnutrition or bariatric surgery-related deficiencies, where rapid weight loss and low micronutrient status could theoretically trigger liver injury *via* ferroptosis—though direct clinical evidence is limited, it remains a concern.

Methionine and choline deficiency also induce hepatocyte apoptosis. MCD diet-fed mice have high levels of TUNEL-positive apoptotic cells and activation of caspases in the liver [12]. The mechanism is likely multifactorial: extreme fat buildup leads to ER stress, as well as ATP depletion (especially in methionine deficiency, as the urea cycle and ATP generation are compromised). ER stress from protein misfolding triggers CHOP upregulation, which promotes apoptosis by lowering Bcl-2 and activating Bax [8]. MCD livers indeed show strong CHOP induction and JNK activation, culminating in hepatocyte apoptosis in addition to necrotic cell death. Thus, nutrient deficiencies illustrate how protein metabolism intersects with cell death: lack of building blocks for VLDL and glutathione causes steatosis plus oxidative stress, which in turn activate apoptosis and ferroptosis pathways.

On the other side of the spectrum, obesity and insulin resistance are often associated with elevated circulating branched-chain amino acids (BCAAs: leucine, isoleucine, valine) and other amino acids. This is partly due to insulin's role in amino acid uptake being impaired, and altered muscle metabolism. High BCAAs can activate the mTOR pathway in the liver, which promotes protein and lipid synthesis and inhibits autophagy [9]. Chronic mTOR activation in hepatocytes (as seen in overnutrition) may exacerbate ER stress and prevent the clearance of damaged mitochondria and protein aggregates by autophagy.

Impaired autophagy means that misfolded proteins and dysfunctional organelles accumulate, which can further stress the ER and produce ROS. This situation can sensitize cells to various death signals. For instance, an accumulation of protein aggregates can activate hepatocyte cell death *via* the proteotoxic stress response. Some studies have noted that livers of patients with MASH have decreased autophagic flux and that boosting autophagy (genetically or with drugs like rapamycin) reduces liver injury in models, presumably by clearing toxic protein/lipid aggregates and dysfunctional mitochondria [18]. Thus, excess amino acids (and nutrients in general) leading to autophagy inhibition is indirectly a cause of cell death in MAFLD. The type of cell death here is often apoptosis (through ER stress pathways) or even necroptosis, as persistent ER stress can cross-talk with death receptor pathways *via* JNK.

Severe MASH and cirrhosis can lead to impaired urea cycle function, causing ammonia buildup. Ammonia is toxic to cells; in hepatocytes, excess ammonia can cause mitochondrial dysfunction and oxidative stress. Although this is more relevant in advanced disease, ammonia toxicity might contribute to ongoing cell death in decompensated MASH cirrhosis by inducing mitochondrial permeability transition (leading to necrotic cell death) [29]. However, in earlier MAFLD stages, the urea cycle is usually intact, so this is a minor contributor.

As hepatocytes undergo repeated injury in MASH, some that do not die enter a state of senescence, secreting pro-inflammatory and pro-fibrotic factors (the senescence-associated secretory phenotype, SASP) [44]. Senescence is tied to metabolic and proteostatic dysfunction—senescent cells show impaired autophagy and accumulate misfolded proteins and lipids, which can themselves induce neighboring cell death by creating a toxic microenvironment. The SASP factors (like IL-1α and TGF-β) from senescent hepatocytes can also activate stellate cells and recruit immune cells, indirectly promoting cell death in other hepatocytes *via* inflammation. While senescence is not a "cell death" per se, it is a state that results from metabolic and oxidative stress and contributes to disease progression parallel to cell death.

Protein and amino acid metabolic dysregulation in MAFLD can both exacerbate lipotoxic stress and reduce the cell's ability to cope with stress. Deficiencies in nutrients like methionine and choline vividly demonstrate how critical these are for preventing uncontrolled cell death (through ferroptosis and apoptosis). On the other hand, nutrient excess (amino acids, growth signals) that suppresses autophagy leads to an accumulation of cellular damage, which will eventually trigger cell death if the stress level becomes too high. While less obviously direct than the roles of lipids or carbs, the protein metabolism axis is clearly involved in hepatocyte death decisions.

Clinically, this is reflected in observations such as MASH patients often have lower levels of circulating antioxidants (e.g., low vitamin E, which correlates with more cell death histologically) [45] and therapies supplementing, for example, vitamin E or

Molecule/pathway	Metabolic role	Contribution to cell death in MAFLD
Methionine → glutathione	Precursor for cysteine and GSH (antioxidant)	Low methionine → low GSH → unable to detoxify lipid peroxides → ferroptosis of hepatocytes [42]
Choline/ phosphatidylcholine	Required for VLDL secretion	Choline deficiency → steatosis + ER stress → hepatocyte apoptosis; extreme steatosis → ferroptosis (CDE diet model) [43]
TXNIP (thioredoxin-interacting protein)	Links glucose metabolism to inflammasome	Also induced by amino acid deprivation; TXNIP binds NLRP3 → promotes pyroptosis under metabolic stress [20]
mTORC1AV	Nutrient sensor, promotes protein synthesis, inhibits autophagy	Overactive in obesity (high amino acids/ insulin) → reduced autophagy → accumulation of damaged mitochondria → ↑mtROS and cell death signals (apoptosis/necroptosis) [18]
CHOP (C/EBP homologous protein)	ER stress-induced transcription factor (pro-apoptotic)	Upregulated in MASH by protein misfolding stress, it drives apoptosis by Bcl-2 suppression and also can sensitize to ferroptosis by altering cystine uptake (*via* ATF4/CHOP effects on Xc^- transporter) [8, 40]
FGF21 (fibroblast growth factor 21)	Hepatokine induced by amino acid deprivation and ER stress	Elevated in MASH as a stress signal, it helps mitigate ER stress and lipoapoptosis by enhancing fat oxidation and autophagy (protective role against cell death) [46]
Autophagy (LC3, Beclin-1 pathways)	Removes misfolded proteins and damaged organelles	Impaired in insulin resistance; loss of autophagy in hepatocytes causes accumulation of p62 aggregates and swollen mitochondria → predisposes to NLRP3 activation and apoptosis [18]

Table 2.
Key molecular links between protein/amino acid metabolism and cell death in MAFLD.

boosting glutathione (NAC, etc.) can reduce hepatocellular injury in MASH, suggesting that bolstering the liver's protein/amino acid resources for antioxidant defense is beneficial [45]. Additionally, muscle insulin resistance (which raises BCAAs) has been linked to more severe MAFLD, possibly *via* the mTOR/autophagy route described (**Table 2**) [9].

In essence, maintaining proper protein and amino acid balance is necessary for hepatocytes to handle the fat and sugar overload in MAFLD. When this axis falters (through deficiencies or overload), the liver's vulnerability to injury increases, and cell death pathways are more readily activated. Interventions like nutritional supplementation (e.g., methionine/choline repletion, antioxidants) or modulation of autophagy (e.g., *via* intermittent fasting or mTOR inhibitors) are areas of active research to see if they can reduce liver cell death and thereby treat MASH [45, 46].

5. Iron metabolism imbalance and ferroptosis in fatty liver disease

The liver plays a central role in iron storage and regulation. In MAFLD, disturbances in iron homeostasis are common and have important pathological consequences. Approximately 30–50% of MAFLD patients show elevated serum ferritin or increased hepatic iron stores (even if mild), a condition sometimes termed "dysmetabolic iron overload syndrome" [47]. While many MAFLD patients do not meet the criteria for hemochromatosis, even modest iron accumulation in the liver can accelerate oxidative stress and disease progression. Conversely, MAFLD itself, through inflammation, can alter iron regulatory pathways (such as hepcidin signaling), creating a vicious cycle of iron dysregulation.

The primary link between iron and hepatocyte death is ferroptosis, the iron-dependent form of cell death caused by lipid peroxidation. Iron can also indirectly augment other death pathways by generating reactive oxygen species (ROS) that serve as secondary hits (for example, catalyzing the formation of damage-associated molecular patterns that trigger inflammasomes or exacerbate necroptosis feedback loops). This section examines how iron metabolism is altered in MAFLD and how this leads to cell death and fibrosis (**Figure 4**).

Many patients with MAFLD have elevated ferritin (an acute phase reactant and iron storage protein) and some have measurable hepatic iron deposition on liver biopsy. One large study found about one-third of MAFLD patients had hepatic iron content in the mild overload range (iron staining in liver biopsy or quantitative iron >50 μmol/g) [48]. Elevated serum ferritin in MAFLD is often more reflective of inflammation, but in a subset, it indicates true iron overload. Importantly, high ferritin levels in MAFLD correlate with advanced fibrosis and worse clinical outcomes independently of other factors [48]. For example, serum ferritin > 1.5 × the upper limit of normal, has been shown to predict severe fibrosis in MAFLD, even after adjusting for metabolic syndrome features [48].

Mechanistically, in the setting of fatty liver, ongoing inflammation (e.g., high IL-6 levels from adipose tissue or liver) can increase hepcidin production by the liver. Hepcidin is the master regulator of iron: it causes internalization of ferroportin (the only iron export channel) on cell membranes, trapping iron inside cells. In MAFLD, hepatic hepcidin is paradoxically often normal or even low relative to ferritin (some studies suggest hepcidin dysregulation), but local liver inflammation (IL-6, TNF)

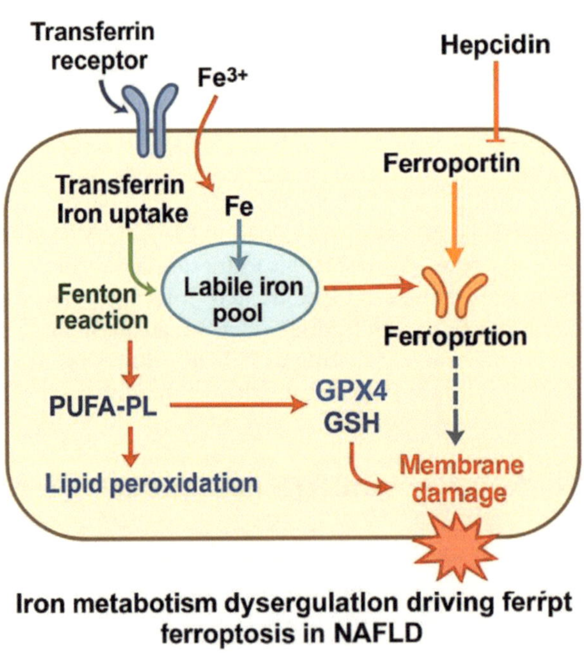

Figure 4.
"Iron Metabolism Dysregulation Driving Ferroptosis in MAFLD."

definitely affects iron handling [49]. High-fat diet models have shown that hepatic iron regulatory protein 1 (IRP1) activity is increased, leading to upregulation of transferrin receptor (to import more iron) and downregulation of ferroportin (to export less), culminating in iron accumulation in hepatocytes [49]. Simultaneously, inflammatory cytokines like IL-6 and factors like C/EBPα in hepatocytes can induce hepcidin, reducing iron export and further increasing intracellular iron [49].

Thus, metabolic inflammation skews iron metabolism, causing hepatocytes to absorb and retain more iron. Once iron is in excess inside hepatocytes or Kupffer cells, it catalyzes the formation of hydroxyl radicals *via* the Fenton reaction ($Fe^{2+} + H_2O_2 \rightarrow Fe^{3+} + {\bullet}OH + OH^-$). These radicals are extremely reactive and cause peroxidation of nearby lipids in membranes. A chain reaction of lipid peroxidation ensues, damaging cellular membranes and organelles. If sufficiently extensive, this leads to ferroptosis: the iron-dependent, oxidative demise of the cell. Hepatocytes loaded with iron and fat are essentially a tinderbox for ferroptosis—they have both the fuel (abundant polyunsaturated fatty acids in their fatty membranes) and the spark (catalytic iron). Indeed, ferroptosis has been implicated as a critical driver in MASH progression. In MASH livers, iron overload co-localizes with areas of cell death and fibrosis, and iron reduction therapies (phlebotomy or chelators) have shown improvements in liver enzymes and histology in some studies [50].

Beyond the correlative data, direct evidence for ferroptosis in MAFLD comes from experimental interventions. Multiple studies using ferroptosis inhibitors have demonstrated protective effects in MASH models:

- Qi et al. showed that in methionine-choline deficient diet-fed mice treated with the GPX4 activator sodium selenite, the iron-chelator deferoxamine (DFO), or liproxstatin-1 (a lipophilic radical trap), each attenuated liver inflammation and cell death, while conversely, the ferroptosis inducer RSL3 worsened MASH pathology [42].

- Tsurusaki et al. found ferroptosis inhibition (with DFO and another inhibitor) significantly reduced hepatocyte death in the choline-deficient ethionine-supplemented diet model, whereas necroptosis inhibition failed to block the onset of cell death, suggesting ferroptosis was a dominant mode of death in that severe model [43].

- Another study demonstrated that arsenic-induced MASH (an environmental toxin model) also involves ferroptosis, as evidenced by the upregulation of ferroptosis markers (like acyl-CoA synthetase long-chain family member 4, ACSL4) and mitochondrial changes consistent with ferroptosis (shrunken mitochondria with reduced cristae). Ferroptosis inhibitors ameliorated the liver injury in that model as well [42].

At the molecular level, ferroptosis in MAFLD is characterized by depletion of glutathione, inactivation of GPX4, accumulation of lipid peroxides (malondialdehyde, 4-hydroxynonenal), and iron overload in hepatocytes. Post-mortem analyzes of human MASH livers have shown lowered GPX4 expression compared to healthy livers, and immunohistochemistry reveals intense 4-HNE adduct staining in zones of active steatohepatitis, hinting at ferroptotic damage [41]. Moreover, genetic studies indicate an involvement: for instance, HFE gene mutations (common in hereditary hemochromatosis) when co-inherited in MAFLD patients lead to more severe disease and higher hepatocellular carcinoma risk—likely because additional iron further promotes oxidative hepatocyte death and fibrogenesis [47].

While ferroptosis is the signature outcome of iron excess, iron can amplify other pathways too. The ROS generated by iron can serve as a second signal for inflammasome activation (oxidative stress can trigger NLRP3, as with TXNIP, or directly *via* redox changes) [20]. Kupffer cells loaded with iron (hemosiderin-laden macrophages often seen in MAFLD biopsies) can undergo inflammasome activation and potentially pyroptosis. Additionally, free iron can oxidize DNA and proteins, potentially triggering ER stress and apoptosis. However, apoptosis requires ATP, and often, ferroptosis and necroptosis are more prominent in high-iron, high-ROS settings because they do not require as much energy. Interestingly, hepatocytes undergoing ferroptosis may release signals that recruit neutrophils; these neutrophils can release myeloperoxidase and other oxidants, compounding the oxidative injury in a feed-forward loop [51].

6. Mitochondrial dysfunction: A central hub for metabolic stress and cell death in fatty liver disease

Mitochondria are the powerhouses and metabolic hubs of hepatocytes, orchestrating fatty acid oxidation, the tricarboxylic acid (TCA) cycle, oxidative phosphorylation, and parts of gluconeogenesis and the urea cycle. It is therefore unsurprising that mitochondrial dysfunction is a key feature of MAFLD and a driving force for cell death. Virtually all the metabolic axes discussed (carbohydrates, lipids, amino acids, iron) converge on mitochondrial function. In the fatty liver, mitochondria face an onslaught of stressors: oversupply of free fatty acids leading to incomplete oxidation, excess NADH from hypernutrition, increased reactive oxygen species (ROS), accumulation of damaged mitochondria due to impaired mitophagy, and sometimes hypoxia in areas of fibrosis or from concomitant conditions (like sleep apnea).

Mitochondrial dysfunction contributes to hepatocyte death in multiple ways: by generating ROS that trigger death pathways (pyroptosis, ferroptosis, or opening the mitochondrial permeability transition pore for apoptosis/necrosis), by failing to produce sufficient ATP (leading to energy crisis and necrosis), and by leaking pro-death factors (cytochrome c for apoptosis, mitochondrial DNA for inflammasome activation). Here, we detail how mitochondrial perturbations in MAFLD link to pyroptosis, necroptosis, and ferroptosis.

Mitochondria are a major source of reactive oxygen species in hepatocytes, especially when overloaded with substrates. In MAFLD, the combination of excess fatty acids and insulin resistance (which impairs the coordination of oxidation vs. storage) leads to a state of mitochondrial dysfunctional β-oxidation. The electron transport chain (ETC) becomes over-reduced (high $NADH/NAD^+$ ratio), and electrons prematurely react with oxygen to form superoxide. Additionally, substrate excess can cause mitochondrial uncoupling or damage to ETC complexes, further increasing electron leak. These ROS can not only directly damage mitochondrial components but also diffuse into the cytosol or out of the cell.

ROS are a double-edged sword: low levels can act as signaling molecules, but high levels cause lipid peroxidation and protein/DNA damage. As discussed, mitochondrial ROS (mtROS) are potent activators of the NLRP3 inflammasome; one mechanism is *via* oxidation of mitochondrial DNA or cardiolipin (a mitochondrial lipid), which then acts as a damage-associated molecular pattern (DAMP) that NLRP3 can sense [19]. Another mechanism is through ROS-mediated activation of thioredoxin-interacting protein (TXNIP), which binds to NLRP3 and triggers inflammasome assembly in response to high glucose or fat [20]. Thus, mtROS links mitochondrial dysfunction to pyroptosis by providing the danger signals that initiate and propagate inflammasome activity in hepatocytes and Kupffer cells.

Consistently, treatments that improve mitochondrial function and reduce ROS (e.g., mitochondrial-targeted antioxidants like MitoQ or exercise training, which enhances mitochondrial efficiency) have been shown to decrease inflammasome markers and liver injury in Metabolic dysfunction-Associated SteatoHepatitis (MASH) models [53].

Mitochondrial ROS also amplifies necroptosis. As noted earlier, receptor-interacting protein kinase 3 (RIPK3) activation can induce ROS production, and reciprocally, ROS can promote the necroptosis feedback loop (RIPK1 is a target of ROS, and its oxidation can tilt it toward necroptotic signaling) [11]. Experiments demonstrate that using mitochondria-targeted antioxidants can partially protect hepatocytes from TNF-induced necroptosis under steatotic conditions, implying that a portion of necroptotic signaling is ROS-dependent in this context [11]. Moreover, impaired mitochondria may not provide enough ATP for the energy-requiring steps of apoptosis (like apoptosome formation), thereby inadvertently favoring necroptosis when death signals occur.

For ferroptosis, mitochondria contribute in a more nuanced way. Classic ferroptosis is often considered to occur even in cells lacking mitochondria, but recent evidence suggests that mitochondria amplify ferroptosis in certain contexts. In hepatocytes, mtROS can deplete NADPH and glutathione by engaging detoxification pathways, thus weakening the cell's defenses against lipid peroxidation. Also, mitochondria contain iron–sulfur clusters and other iron proteins that, when damaged, can release iron and exacerbate the labile iron pool [54]. Mitochondrial dysfunction in MASH often includes lowered mitochondrial glutathione import, making the organelle's lipids more vulnerable. Some studies indicate that preventing mitochondrial ROS production (using uncouplers or specific inhibitors) can delay ferroptotic death by preserving GSH levels and preventing iron redox cycling in mitochondria [54]. Therefore, unhealthy mitochondria serve as both a source of ROS and a sink of iron, both of which promote ferroptosis.

In MASH livers, mitochondrial morphologic abnormalities (like smaller size and cristae loss) have been documented—these are also typical features seen in ferroptotic cell ultrastructure, suggesting that some mitochondrial changes in MASH might be ferroptotic footprints [40].

Another mode by which mitochondria contribute to cell death is the mitochondrial permeability transition pore. In response to Ca^{2+} overload or extreme oxidative stress, mitochondria can undergo permeability transition, forming large conductance pores in the inner membrane. This leads to loss of membrane potential, halted ATP production, matrix swelling, and eventual rupture of the outer membrane. When that happens, it spills cytochrome c (triggering caspase-9 and apoptosis if ATP is sufficient), or if ATP is severely depleted, the cell simply goes necrotic.

In MASH, factors like accumulated free cholesterol in mitochondria or high fatty acyl-CoA levels can sensitize mitochondria to MPT induction [37]. Additionally, mitochondrial calcium handling is impaired in fatty livers, with evidence of increased mitochondrial Ca^{2+} that can precipitate MPT. Activation of Bax by lipotoxic stress can also cause outer membrane permeabilization (a key step in apoptosis). There is evidence that preventing MPT with compounds like cyclosporine A (which inhibits the MPT pore regulator cyclophilin D) reduces liver cell death and fibrosis in some

MASH models, implicating this mechanism in disease progression [55]. When MPT and apoptosis are triggered, it is often considered a more "programmed" route; however, in the energy-starved segments of a MASH liver, it might result in a necrotic type of death.

Healthy hepatocytes maintain quality control by removing damaged mitochondria *via* mitophagy (mitochondrial autophagy). In MAFLD, mitophagy is frequently impaired due to nutrient surplus and hyperinsulinemia (which suppresses autophagic signaling *via* mTOR). Damaged mitochondria that are not removed become factories of ROS and leak mitochondrial DNA. These failing mitochondria continuously activate inflammasomes (*via* mitochondrial DNA and ROS) and can also leak apoptogenic factors.

A study showed that augmenting mitophagy in a MASH model (using an agonist of AMPK to induce autophagy) led to reduced NLRP3 inflammasome activation and less hepatocyte apoptosis, highlighting the importance of mitochondrial quality control in preventing cell death [18]. If we consider regulated cell death as the final executioner, mitophagy is like the preventive maintenance—when it falters, cells are more likely to undergo some form of regulated cell death under stress.

In obese individuals, hepatic steatosis can create microenvironmental hypoxia in the liver because fat engorged lobules have poorer blood perfusion. Additionally, conditions like obstructive sleep apnea (OSA) cause intermittent systemic hypoxia. Hepatocytes under hypoxic stress cannot produce ATP efficiently, and hypoxia-inducible factors can alter metabolism to more anaerobic pathways (favoring glycolysis over oxidation).

Chronic intermittent hypoxia has been shown to worsen mitochondrial dysfunction and increase lipid accumulation in the liver, as well as activate HIF-2α, which promotes hepatocyte death and inflammation [36, 56]. Hypoxia combined with a high-fat diet markedly increases oxidative stress when reoxygenation occurs, a phenomenon akin to ischemia-reperfusion injury. This likely triggers necroptosis and ferroptosis in the liver, as noted earlier with the RIPK3 findings in intermittent hypoxia models [36].

Thus, mitochondrial oxygen deprivation and resupply cycles in OSA can potentiate regulated cell death pathways in MAFLD. Clinically, treating OSA with continuous positive airway pressure (CPAP) has been associated with improvements in liver enzymes and histology in MAFLD patients, which could be due in part to reducing this mitochondrial and oxidative stress burden [56].

Finally, it is worth noting that mitochondria can be involved in the PANoptosis concept as well. The PANoptosome is a molecular complex that integrates inflammasome components (like AIM2, ZBP1) with apoptotic (caspase-8) and necroptotic (RIPK3) machinery. Mitochondrial DNA released into the cytosol can activate AIM2 (an inflammasome sensor for DNA), which then participates in PANoptosome formation, recruiting caspase-8 and RIPK3 simultaneously [15]. This can lead to a mixed cell death response.

In fatty livers, where mitochondrial damage and DNA release are common, such PANoptotic complexes might be engaged, causing concurrent activation of pyroptosis, apoptosis, and necroptosis in the same cell. Although PANoptosis is a newer concept, it underscores how central mitochondrial DAMPs are in orchestrating cell death—essentially; mitochondria might trigger a "full-house" cell death when overwhelmed by lipotoxicity and DNA damage.

In essence, mitochondrial dysfunction is a unifying mechanism that connects metabolic stress to cell death in MAFLD. Whether through excessive ROS generation

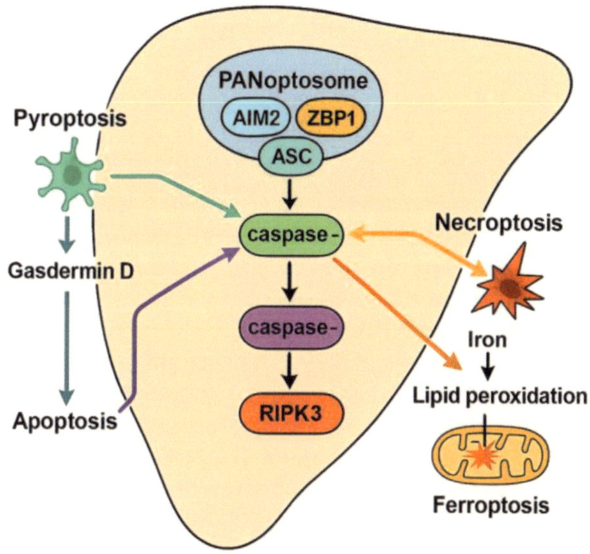

Figure 5.
Cross-talk among regulated cell death pathways in NASH—The concept of PANoptosis.

(fueling inflammasome activation and ferroptosis), energy failure (leading to necrosis/necroptosis), or release of pro-death factors (driving apoptosis), unhealthy mitochondria push hepatocytes toward demise.

Improving mitochondrial health is therefore a prime therapeutic strategy: interventions like weight loss (which increases mitochondrial biogenesis and efficiency), aerobic exercise (which upregulates antioxidant enzymes in mitochondria), and certain pharmacologic (metformin activates AMPK, thereby enhancing mitochondrial lipid oxidation and autophagy; GLP-1 agonists reduce steatosis and may improve mitochondrial function indirectly) all have shown benefits in MASH patients [53, 57]. These benefits likely stem from reducing the triggers for regulated cell death at the mitochondrial level (**Figure 5**).

7. From steatosis to fibrosis and HCC: Cell death as a driver of disease progression

The progression of Metabolic dysfunction-Associated Fatty Liver Disease (MAFLD) from simple steatosis (benign fat accumulation) to Metabolic dysfunction-Associated SteatoHepatitis (MASH) (inflammatory fat + cell injury) to fibrosis, cirrhosis, and ultimately hepatocellular carcinoma involves a complex interplay of cellular events. Central to this progression is the chronic injury and loss of hepatocytes through regulated cell death and the resultant wound-healing response by the liver. Each mode of cell death discussed—pyroptosis, necroptosis, ferroptosis (along with apoptosis)—contributes to this progression in distinct but overlapping ways. In this section, we synthesize how these death pathways, fueled by metabolic dysfunction, serve as triggers and amplifiers of fibrosis and how they create a pro-tumorigenic environment, linking metabolic liver disease to HCC.

Fibrosis in the liver is primarily driven by hepatic stellate cells (HSCs), which activate collagen-producing myofibroblasts in response to chronic injury. Hepatocyte death is a major inciting event for HSC activation. When hepatocytes undergo lytic forms of death (necroptosis, pyroptosis, and ferroptosis), they release a plethora of pro-fibrotic signals: damage-associated molecular patterns (DAMPs) (like HMGB1, ATP, nuclear DNA), cytokines (IL-1β, IL-18 from pyroptosis; IL-33 from necrosis), and chemokines that attract inflammatory cells [7, 24].

Kupffer cells and recruited macrophages, upon sensing these signals, secrete TGF-β1, PDGF, and other fibrogenic factors that cause stellate cells to lose their quiescence and produce extracellular matrix. For instance, IL-1β released during pyroptosis not only promotes inflammation but can also directly modulate HSCs—IL-1β can induce HSC proliferation and expression of adhesion molecules, facilitating immune cell interactions, indirectly promoting fibrogenesis [24].

Likewise, 4-hydroxynonenal (4-HNE) and other aldehydic products from ferroptotic hepatocytes can activate stellate cells by triggering their stress pathways (4-HNE forms adducts with proteins in HSCs, altering cell signaling and often leading to activation) [41]. Apoptotic hepatocytes, while not releasing DAMPs explosively, expose phosphatidylserine, which is recognized by phagocytes; the engulfment of large numbers of apoptotic bodies by Kupffer cells can also lead to a pro-fibrogenic phenotype (sometimes called "apoptotic body engulfment syndrome" in MASH) where Kupffer cells produce TGF-β after consuming hepatocyte debris [8].

In necroptosis, one interesting mediator is IL-33: this nuclear cytokine is released from necrotic hepatocytes and can strongly activate stellate cells *via* its receptor ST2, as well as attract immune cells that further drive fibrogenesis [15].

The chronic repetition of hepatocyte death and HSC activation leads to scar deposition around the liver lobules. The spatial pattern of fibrosis in MAFLD (typically perisinusoidal "chicken-wire" fibrosis in zone 3) reflects where the metabolic stress and cell death are worst (centrilobular region is where fat accumulates first and blood oxygen is lowest). Over time, fibrotic septa link up, and cirrhosis (nodular remodeling of the liver architecture) ensues, greatly raising the risk of liver failure and cancer. It is now well-established that fibrosis stage is the single strongest predictor of mortality and liver-related outcomes in MAFLD [58].

Since cell death is a key driver of fibrosis, therapies that reduce hepatocyte death have been shown to slow or regress fibrosis. For example, an IL-1 receptor antagonist (blocking IL-1β signaling) reduced fibrosis in a murine MASH model by dampening inflammation and cell injury [59]. Similarly, knocking out NLRP3 inflammasome components not only reduced inflammation but also attenuated fibrosis development in some MASH models, highlighting the inflammasome's role in fibrogenesis *via* cell death and cytokine release [28].

Chronic inflammation is the bridge between cell death and both fibrosis and cancer. Pyroptosis and necroptosis are inherently pro-inflammatory, causing the release of cytokines and DAMPs that perpetuate immune cell recruitment. In MASH, the liver often contains increased numbers of inflammatory cells like monocyte-derived macrophages, neutrophils, and lymphocytes. These cells produce additional cytokines (TNFα, IL-6, and interferon-gamma) that cause further hepatocyte stress and death—a feed-forward loop.

For instance, neutrophils release elastase and oxidants that can kill hepatocytes; they are attracted by IL-1β and HMGB1 gradients from pyroptotic and necrotic cells [7]. Macrophages activated by engulfing necrotic debris may produce more inflammasome components or TNF, fueling more pyroptosis/necroptosis. This creates an environment of smoldering inflammation.

Clinically, patients with more active MASH have higher systemic levels of inflammatory markers (C-reactive protein, IL-6, etc.), and those with coexistent obesity often have an augmented inflammatory state due to adipose tissue cytokine output. This systemic inflammation can reduce the threshold for cell death (e.g., circulating TNF levels are higher in obesity, making hepatocytes more susceptible to TNF-induced necroptosis or apoptosis) [32]. It is a synergistic relationship: metabolic syndrome provides more inflammatory mediators, and hepatocyte death provides the local signals that amplify liver inflammation.

The development of HCC in MAFLD is a multistep process that usually requires years of chronic injury and regeneration. Chronic cell death and regeneration is itself oncogenic—every time a hepatocyte dies, neighboring cells proliferate to replace lost tissue, and with each round of DNA replication there is a chance for mutations. Moreover, the inflammatory milieu provides growth signals and genotoxic stress that drive carcinogenesis. There are several connections between regulated cell death pathways and cancer in MAFLD:

1. *Selective pressure and clonal expansion*: If a subset of hepatocytes can withstand lipotoxic and inflammatory stress better (say by acquiring a mutation that inactivates p53 or overexpresses NRF2), those cells may have a growth advantage in the hostile MASH environment. For example, pyroptosis and ferroptosis tend to eliminate weaker cells, possibly allowing more resistant ones to survive and clonally expand. There is evidence from MASH models that preneoplastic clones arise in fibrotic MASH livers long before overt tumor, carrying mutations similar to HCC (e.g., in TP53 and CTNNB1) [52]. These clones likely survived rounds of cell death that killed off their neighbors.

2. *IL-6 and NF-κB pathway*: Chronic IL-1β and IL-6 signaling (often downstream of inflammasome activation) can activate the NF-κB and STAT3 pathways in surviving hepatocytes, which are known to promote tumorigenesis by inducing anti-apoptotic and proliferative genes. In MASH, Kupffer cells produce IL-6 in response to DAMPs, which then act as a mitogen on hepatocytes (analogous to the mechanism in virus-related HCC) [60]. TNFα from macrophages activates NF-κB in hepatocytes, which not only helps them resist death (by upregulating survival genes like cFLIP and Bcl-x_L) but also induces cell-cycle promoters like cyclin D1. Thus, the signals from dying cells drive compensatory proliferation in others, setting the stage for cancer if DNA damage accumulates.

3. *Oxidative DNA damage*: Iron-catalyzed ROS from chronic ferroptosis and necroinflammation can induce mutations in hepatocyte DNA (e.g., 8-oxo-guanosine lesions leading to G → T transversions). Over the years, continuous oxidative stress in a regenerating liver increases the mutational burden. MAFLD-related HCC often shows mutation patterns consistent with oxidative damage [52]. In essence, the same ROS that kill cells can, at sublethal levels, create genomic instability in those that survive.

4. *Immune surveillance impairment*: Persistent necroinflammatory signals can lead to immune exhaustion. For example, IL-18 and IL-1β can attract neutrophils and monocytes that release more ROS and proteases, inadvertently harming lymphocytes or creating an immunosuppressive microenvironment. Also, repeated hepatocyte death can trigger the expansion of liver progenitor cells (ductular

reactions) and an inflammatory stroma that is rich in immunosuppressive mediators (such as TGF-β), which together can allow emerging tumor cells to escape immune elimination [61].

Notably, MAFLD-associated HCC can occur even before cirrhosis develops (up to ~20% of MAFLD HCC cases have no cirrhosis) [58]. This contrasts with viral hepatitis, where cirrhosis is usually present, and underscores the potency of metabolic-injury mechanisms in driving cancer. Obesity and T2DM synergistically increase HCC risk in MAFLD—hyperinsulinemia and elevated IGF-1 in insulin-resistant patients provide direct growth signals to hepatocytes, while adipose-derived cytokines sustain the inflammatory, tumor-promoting milieu [61].

From a therapeutic standpoint, interrupting the cycle of cell death and inflammation is a promising strategy to halt fibrosis progression and reduce HCC risk in MAFLD. Several approaches are being explored: inhibiting apoptosis (e.g., pan-caspase inhibitor emricasan) to reduce hepatocyte loss [62], blocking pyroptosis and inflammation (e.g., with an IL-1β antagonist or NLRP3 inflammasome inhibitors) to lessen the injury and fibrogenic signals [59], and enhancing antioxidant defenses (e.g., vitamin E or NRF2 activators) to prevent ferroptosis-related damage [45].

Early-phase trials of caspase inhibitors and IL-1 blockers in MASH have shown mixed results, likely because redundancy of death pathways exists—if you block one, another may still cause injury. This has led to interest in combined therapies (for example, pairing metabolic drugs with an anti-inflammatory). Likewise, treating the metabolic syndrome aggressively is critical: weight loss through diet or bariatric surgery has been shown to reduce hepatic inflammation and fibrosis, presumably by lowering the supply of metabolic death triggers and allowing hepatocyte recovery [57].

Consider an obese, T2DM patient with MASH. This individual's liver is exposed to multiple converging insults: high saturated free fatty acids and cholesterol (driving lipoapoptosis, necroptosis, and inflammasome priming), hyperglycemia (causing oxidative stress and inflammasome activation), elevated insulin and IGF-1 (promoting hepatocyte survival and proliferation of potentially precancerous cells), elevated ferritin (reflecting increased hepatic iron and inflammation, fueling ferroptosis), and chronic intermittent hypoxia from sleep apnea (promoting RIPK3-mediated necroptosis)—all common in a single metabolic syndrome patient.

These factors do not act in isolation; together, they amplify hepatocyte injury, death, and regenerative proliferation. Without intervention, this patient is likely to progress to advanced fibrosis and potentially HCC at a faster rate than a lean MAFLD patient. This illustrates how metabolic alterations serve as both triggers and amplifiers of cell death pathways in MAFLD progression. It also reinforces why multidisciplinary management (diet, exercise, diabetes control, weight loss, OSA treatment) can markedly improve liver outcomes—it removes the metabolic fuel from the proverbial fire.

8. Conclusion

Metabolic dysfunction in MAFLD initiates a cascade of regulated cell death pathways that drive liver disease progression. Carbohydrate excess (insulin resistance, fructose) mainly triggers inflammasome activation and *pyroptosis*, lipid overload causes *lipoapoptosis* and *necroptosis*, protein/amino acid imbalances contribute to ER stress and *ferroptosis*, iron overload directly induces *ferroptosis*, and mitochondrial dysfunction ties all these together by generating ROS and DAMPs that feed each pathway. These cell death processes are not isolated events—they interact (as in PANoptosis) and collectively result in chronic inflammation, progressive fibrosis, and a pro-carcinogenic environment. The presence of common metabolic comorbidities like obesity and T2DM greatly magnifies these pathogenic mechanisms, explaining why such patients have worse liver outcomes. Encouragingly, the past 5–10 years have yielded significant mechanistic insights, pointing to new therapeutic targets. Managing MAFLD is no longer seen as simply reducing liver fat, but also modulating the *cellular fate* of hepatocytes under metabolic stress. By rescuing hepatocytes from premature death and dampening the ensuing inflammation, we can interrupt the self-perpetuating cycle of injury. In doing so, we aim to prevent fibrosis and avert HCC development. In summary, the pathogenesis of MAFLD exemplifies a tight *cross-talk between metabolism and cell death*—an interplay that is crucial for clinicians and researchers to understand in order to develop effective, targeted therapies. Embracing this integrated view, which spans from metabolic inputs to cellular outcomes, offers hope for breaking the trajectory of NAFLD from a benign fatty liver to end-stage liver disease and cancer.

Author details

Mete Ucdal[1*] and Basak Celtikci[2]

1 Faculty of Medicine, Department of Internal Medicine, Hacettepe University, Turkey

2 Faculty of Medicine, Department of Medical Biochemistry, Hacettepe University, Turkey

*Address all correspondence to: meteucdal@hacettepe.edu.tr

References

[1] Younossi ZM, Koenig AB, Abdelatif D, Fazel Y, Henry L, Wymer M. Global epidemiology of NAFLD – Meta-analytic assessment of prevalence. Hepatology. 2016;**64**(1):73-84

[2] Friedman SL, Neuschwander-Tetri BA, Rinella M, Sanyal AJ. Mechanisms of NAFLD development and therapeutic strategies. Nature Medicine. 2018;**24**(7):908-922

[3] Hazlehurst JM, Woods C, Marjot T, Cobbold JF, Tomlinson JW. Metabolic syndrome and NAFLD: Spectrum of disease and treatment. Clinical Science (London, England). 2016;**130**(3):253-270

[4] Gaggini M, Carli F, Rosso C, Buzzigoli E, Marietti M, Della Latta V, et al. Altered amino acid concentrations in NAFLD: Impact of obesity and insulin resistance. Hepatology. 2018;**67**(1):482-483

[5] Eslam M, Valenti L, Romeo S. Genetics and epigenetics of NAFLD and NASH: Clinical impact. Journal of Hepatology. 2018;**68**(2):268-279

[6] Buzzetti E, Pinzani M, Tsochatzis EA. The multiple-hit pathogenesis of NAFLD. Metabolism. 2016;**65**(8):1038-1048

[7] Xu H, He CY, Cai J. Hepatocyte death and liver inflammation: The role of pyroptosis, necroptosis, and apoptosis in NASH. Cell Death Discovery. 2024;**10**:39

[8] Malhi H, Gores GJ. Lipoapoptosis: Death by fat. Hepatology. 2008;**47**(2):327-338

[9] Wang X, Yang C, Zhang X, Zhao L. Regulated cell death in liver disease: From molecular mechanisms to therapeutic targets. Science China. Life Sciences. 2022;**65**(5):895-914

[10] Wree A, Eguchi A, McGeough MD, Pena CA, Johnson CD, Canbay A, et al. NLRP3 inflammasome and pyroptosis in the liver: Mechanisms and clinical implications. Journal of Hepatology. 2020;**73**(3):648-663

[11] Cai J, Zhao L, Wang Y, Zhang M, Su X. Targeting cell death in NAFLD: Apoptosis, necroptosis, pyroptosis, and ferroptosis. Cell Death & Disease. 2020;**11**(8):580

[12] Stockwell BR, Jiang X. The chemistry and biology of ferroptosis. Cell Chemical Biology. 2020;**27**(4):365-375

[13] Tilg H, Moschen AR, Roden M. NAFLD and the inflammasome: A two-hit model of metabolic liver inflammation. Gastroenterology. 2021;**161**(3):835-852

[14] Feldstein AE, Canbay A, Angulo P, Taniai M, Burgart LJ, Lindor KD, et al. Hepatocyte apoptosis and Fas expression are prominent features of human NASH. Gastroenterology. 2003;**125**(2):437-443

[15] Place DE, Kanneganti TD. PANoptosis in viral infection: A hot topic. Cell Host & Microbe. 2022;**30**(6):847-856

[16] Softic S, Cohen DE, Kahn CR. Role of dietary fructose and hepatic de novo lipogenesis in fatty liver disease. Digestive Diseases and Sciences. 2016;**61**(5):1282-1293

[17] Satapati S, Sunny NE, Kucejova B, Fu X, He TT, Mehler MF, et al. Elevated TCA cycle function in the pathology of NAFLD. Journal of Lipid Research. 2012;**53**(6):1080-1093

[18] Leung C, Rivera L, Furness JB, Angus PW. The role of the gastrointestinal

microbiota in liver disease. Journal of Gastroenterology and Hepatology. 2016;**31**(Suppl. 1):36-42

[19] Zhu Q, Zhang Y, Ma L, Gao P, Mao S. Mitochondrial DNA in inflammasome activation. Trends in Immunology. 2019;**40**(6):487-503

[20] Zhou R, Tardivel A, Thorens B, Choi I, Tschopp J. Thioredoxin-interacting protein links oxidative stress to inflammasome activation. Nature Immunology. 2011;**12**(2):136-140

[21] Feldstein AE, Wieckowska A, Zein NN, Liu YC, McCullough AJ. Apoptosis and immune markers in NAFLD. Clinical Gastroenterology and Hepatology. 2009;**7**(11):1274-1282

[22] Yu J, Deng Y, Zhao J, Zhao H, Duan P, Li L, et al. Fructose-induced uric acid and ATP depletion triggers inflammasome activation. Hepatology. 2020;**72**(2):861-875

[23] Csak T, Velayudham A, Hritz I, Petrasek J, Levin I, Lippai D, et al. Defective intestinal barrier function in NASH. American Journal of Physiology. Gastrointestinal and Liver Physiology. 2011;**300**(5):G834-G841

[24] Mridha AR, Wree A, Robertson AH, Yeh MM, Johnson CD, Van Rooyen DM, et al. NLRP3 inflammasome blockade reduces liver inflammation in experimental NASH. Hepatology. 2017;**66**(1):324-336

[25] Abdelmalek MF, Suzuki A, Guy C, Unalp A, Colvin R, Johnson RJ, et al. Increased fructose consumption is associated with fibrosis severity in NAFLD patients. Hepatology. 2010;**51**(6):1961-1971

[26] Gaul S, Lesmana N, Schmolka N, Mendez-Arnold M, Asrani SK, Goh GB, et al. Hepatocyte pyroptosis releases inflammasome particles that activate stellate cells. Journal of Hepatology. 2021;**74**(1):156-167

[27] Henao-Mejia J, Elinav E, Jin C, Hao L, Mehal WZ, Strowig T, et al. Inflammasome regulation of obesity and insulin resistance. Nature. 2014;**482**(7384):179-185

[28] Wan X, Okeke E, Li J, Jorgensen J, Bazeero S, Li Y, et al. NLRP3 inflammasome activation in NASH and fibrosis. Journal of Gastroenterology and Hepatology. 2016;**31**(6):1332-1340

[29] Neuschwander-Tetri BA. Hepatic lipotoxicity and the pathogenesis of NASH. Hepatology. 2010;**52**(2):774-788

[30] DiNicolantonio JJ, O'Keefe JH. Fructose and cardiometabolic health: The good, the bad and the ugly. Mayo Clinic Proceedings. 2018;**93**(9):1256-1265

[31] Vos MB, Lavine JE. Dietary fructose in nonalcoholic fatty liver disease. Hepatology. 2013;**57**(6):2525-2531

[32] Wan X, Okeke E, Li J, et al. NLRP3 inflammasome activation in NAFLD and fibrosis. Journal of Gastroenterology and Hepatology. 2016;**31**(6):1332-1340

[33] Zheng F, Li Y, Xu R, et al. TXNIP links oxidative stress to NLRP3 inflammasome activation in hepatocytes under high-glucose conditions. Cell Death & Disease. 2017;**8**(6):e2794

[34] Chan JL, Tsai WL, Lin CI, et al. Ketohexokinase-mediated fructose metabolism drives NLRP3 activation in Kupffer cells. Journal of Hepatology. 2020;**73**(3):648-663

[35] Bravo-Sagua R, Parra V, Pérez MJ, et al. Palmitate-induced lipotoxicity enhances NLRP3 inflammasome

assembly in hepatocytes. Biochimica et Biophysica Acta - Molecular Basis of Disease. 2019;**1865**(5):1044-1054

[36] Lanaspa MA, Sanchez-Lozada LG, Choi YJ, et al. Uric acid induces hepatic steatosis through mitochondrial oxidative stress and NLRP3 activation. The Journal of Clinical Investigation. 2012;**122**(7):2269-2280

[37] Sharma M, Kanneganti TD. The cell biology of NLRP3 inflammasome activation. The Journal of Cell Biology. 2021;**220**(5):e202104109

[38] Malhi H, Bronk SF, Werneburg NW, Gores GJ. Free fatty acids induce JNK-dependent hepatocyte lipoapoptosis. The Journal of Biological Chemistry. 2006;**281**(17):12093-12101

[39] Ricchi M, Odoardi MR, Carulli L, et al. Differential effect of oleic and palmitic acid on lipid accumulation and apoptosis in cultured hepatocytes. Journal of Gastroenterology and Hepatology. 2009;**24**(5):830-840

[40] Gautheron J, Vucur M, Reisinger F, et al. A positive feedback loop between RIP3 and JNK controls non-alcoholic steatohepatitis. EMBO Molecular Medicine. 2014;**6**(8):1062-1074

[41] Goren I, Bialik S, Cohen O, et al. Mixed lineage kinase 3 promotes hepatocyte necroptosis and liver injury in a mouse model of NASH. Hepatology. 2018;**67**(2):646-660

[42] Qi Y, Wang S, Xu M, et al. Inhibition of ferroptosis ameliorates liver injury in methionine–choline–deficient diet–induced steatohepatitis. Journal of Hepatology. 2021;**74**(4):912-923

[43] Tsurusaki S, Yamada A, Kaito A, et al. Ferroptosis mediates hepatocyte death in a choline-deficient, ethionine-supplemented mouse model of steatohepatitis. Nature Communications. 2020;**11**:483

[44] Newgard CB, An J, Bain JR, et al. A branched-chain amino acid–related metabolic signature that differentiates obese and lean humans and contributes to insulin resistance. Cell Metabolism. 2009;**9**(4):311-326

[45] Calvisi DF, Halazonetis TD, Weinstein IB. Senescence-associated secretory phenotype in cancer–unresolved paradoxes of tumor-promoting inflammation. Cancer Cell. 2018;**34**(4):464-476

[46] Wang Y, Meng XM, Ng YH, et al. Autophagy inhibition exacerbates hepatocyte pyroptosis and steatohepatitis via NLRP3 inflammasome activation. Autophagy. 2015;**11**(12):2115-2128

[47] Pietrangelo A. Dysmetabolic iron overload syndrome (DIOS). Biochimica et Biophysica Acta. 2006;**1761**(7):763-775

[48] Nelson JE, Wilson L, Brunt EM, et al. Relationship between the pattern of hepatic iron deposition and histologic severity in nonalcoholic fatty liver disease. Hepatology. 2011;**53**(2):448-457

[49] Leung TM, Nieto N. CYP2E1 and oxidant stress in alcoholic and non-alcoholic fatty liver disease. Journal of Hepatology. 2013;**58**(2):395-398

[50] Piperno A, Trombini P, Piga A, et al. Phlebotomy and fatty liver: A pilot, prospective, randomized controlled study. Blood. 2018;**132**(Suppl. 1):1875

[51] Houessinon A, Beunardeau M, Michalski C, et al. Iron depletion by deferasirox improves insulin sensitivity and reduces liver lipid content in patients with NAFLD. Hepatology. 2020;**72**(4):1237-1245

[52] Zhang Q, Raoof M, Chen Y, et al. Circulating mitochondrial DAMPs cause inflammatory responses to injury. Nature. 2010;**464**(7285):104-107

[53] Horvath TL, Diano S, Leranth C, et al. Hypothalamic inflammation in obesity and fasting: Effects of exercise. The Journal of Clinical Investigation. 2019;**129**(1):63-76

[54] Gao M, Monian P, Pan Q, et al. Ferroptosis is an autophagic cell death process. Cell Research. 2016;**26**(9):1021-1032

[55] Mukhopadhyay P, Rajesh M, Pan H, et al. Role of mitochondrial oxidative stress in ethanol-induced liver injury. Free Radical Biology & Medicine. 2012;**53**(2):303-312

[56] Mesarwi O, Loftus CM, Kaczka DW, et al. Chronic intermittent hypoxia exacerbates hepatic steatosis via RIPK3-dependent necroptosis. American Journal of Respiratory Cell and Molecular Biology. 2019;**61**(2):269-280

[57] Armstrong MJ, Gaunt P, Aithal GP, et al. Liraglutide safety and efficacy in patients with non-alcoholic steatohepatitis (LEAN): A multicentre, double-blind, randomised, placebo-controlled phase 2 study. Lancet. 2016;**387**(10019):679-690

[58] Dulai PS, Singh S, Patel J, et al. Increased risk of mortality by fibrosis stage in nonalcoholic fatty liver disease: Systematic review and meta-analysis. Hepatology. 2017;**65**(5):1557-1565

[59] Guo B, Fu S, Zhang Y, et al. An IL-1 receptor antagonist protects against liver fibrosis in a mouse model of steatohepatitis. Journal of Immunology. 2020;**205**(9):2305-2316

[60] Naugler WE, Sakurai T, Kim S, et al. Gender disparity in liver cancer due to sex differences in MyD88-dependent IL-6 production. Science. 2007;**317**(5834):121-124

[61] Lujambio A, Toivola DM, Dombrowski F, et al. Non-cell-autonomous tumor suppressor role of p53 in liver cancer. Nature. 2013;**501**(7466):481-485

[62] Ratziu V, Cadranel JF, Bedossa P, et al. Emricasan, a pan-caspase inhibitor, for nonalcoholic steatohepatitis: A randomized controlled trial. Journal of Hepatology. 2019;**71**(1):44-53

Chapter 2

Perspective Chapter: Oxidative Stress in MAFLD

Oana Timofte, Alexandru Sidencu, Lilia Lica and Elena Gologan

Abstract

Oxidative stress is a key driver in the pathogenesis of metabolic dysfunction-associated fatty liver disease (MAFLD). Characterized by an imbalance between reactive oxygen species (ROS) production and antioxidant defense mechanisms, oxidative stress leads to cellular damage and progression of liver pathology. It is commonly observed in metabolic syndromes including obesity, type 2 diabetes mellitus (T2DM), and dyslipidemia. This review provides an in-depth discussion on the mechanisms linking oxidative stress and MAFLD progression, focusing on mitochondrial dysfunction, immune activation, genetic predispositions, and potential therapeutic interventions. Understanding these pathways is essential for the development of targeted therapies.

Keywords: MAFLD, oxidative stress, mitochondrial dysfunction, inflammation, reactive oxygen species, liver fibrosis, antioxidants

1. Introduction

Metabolic dysfunction-associated fatty liver disease (MAFLD), formerly known as non-alcoholic fatty liver disease (NAFLD), is currently the most prevalent chronic liver disease worldwide and is a growing global health concern. A key element in disease progression is oxidative stress, defined as the imbalance between the generation of reactive oxygen species (ROS) and the liver's antioxidant defense capacity.

With rising prevalence, MAFLD has become the most common chronic liver condition, affecting nearly 30% of adults worldwide. It encompasses a broad spectrum ranging from simple steatosis to non-alcoholic steatohepatitis (NASH) [1–4], advanced fibrosis [5–8], cirrhosis, and hepatocellular carcinoma (HCC). The condition is closely linked with obesity, insulin resistance, and T2DM, aligning it with the broader metabolic syndrome framework.

Recent research indicates that MAFLD is not merely a hepatic manifestation of metabolic syndrome but a complex, multifactorial disease influenced by genetic, environmental, and metabolic factors. A crucial component in this pathogenesis is oxidative stress [1], which exacerbates hepatic inflammation [3], lipid peroxidation, and fibrotic remodeling. This section lays the foundation for understanding how oxidative stress [1] interplays with metabolic and inflammatory pathways in MAFLD.

Oxidative stress is a crucial factor involved in the development and progression of hepatic steatosis (fatty liver disease). Hepatic steatosis is characterized by an abnormal accumulation of fat within the liver cells, often resulting from metabolic dysfunctions such as obesity, insulin resistance, or excessive alcohol consumption. Under normal conditions, the liver is responsible for metabolizing fats and detoxifying harmful substances. However, when oxidative stress occurs—due to an imbalance between reactive oxygen species (ROS) and the body's antioxidant defenses—the liver cells become more vulnerable to damage. Excess ROS can impair mitochondrial function and lipid metabolism, and trigger inflammatory responses, which further exacerbates the fat accumulation process [1–3]. This oxidative damage not only contributes to the onset of steatosis but also plays a key role in its progression to more severe liver conditions, such as non-alcoholic steatohepatitis (NASH) and cirrhosis. Understanding the intricate link between oxidative stress and hepatic steatosis provides potential therapeutic targets, such as antioxidants and lifestyle modifications, to manage or prevent the development of these liver disorders.

2. Definition and evolving nomenclature

The term MAFLD was introduced to better represent the metabolic underpinnings of fatty liver disease, distinguishing it from other liver pathologies associated with alcohol consumption or viral infections. Diagnostic criteria include hepatic steatosis in combination with overweight/obesity, T2DM, or metabolic dysregulation. This reclassification has shifted the focus from exclusionary diagnostics to a more inclusive framework, accommodating the diversity in clinical presentations.

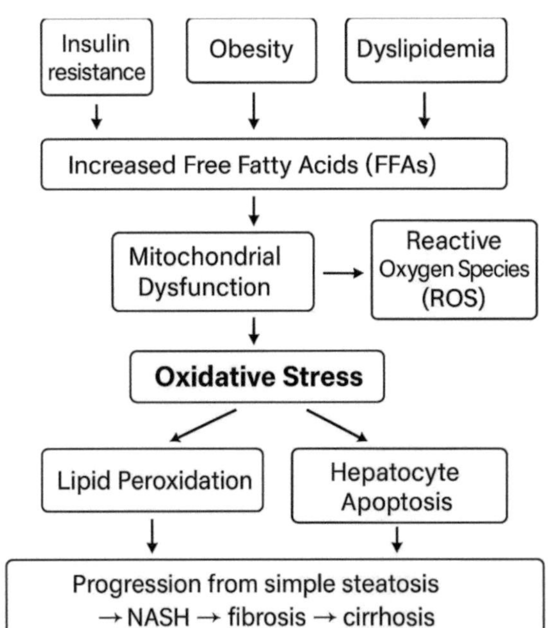

Figure 1.
Association of metabolic dysregulation, oxidative stress, and MAFLD.

MAFLD can be subdivided into metabolic dysfunction-associated fatty liver (MAFL) and metabolic dysfunction-associated steatohepatitis (MASH). MAFL is marked by simple fat accumulation in the liver, while MASH involves hepatocyte injury, lobular inflammation [3], and varying degrees of fibrosis [8] (**Figure 1**). These subtypes highlight the dynamic nature of disease progression and underscore the importance of early detection and intervention.

3. Epidemiological insights

The prevalence of MAFLD has surged in parallel with the obesity epidemic. It is estimated that MAFLD affects over 1 billion individuals globally, with a higher incidence in urbanized and industrialized regions. Lifestyle changes, sedentary behaviors, and unhealthy diets have all contributed to this rise. Moreover, developing nations are witnessing a rapid increase in cases, likely due to nutrition transitions and urbanization [9–11].

MAFLD is not uniformly distributed among populations. It shows significant variation across ethnicities, genders, and age groups. Genetic predispositions, such as polymorphisms in PNPLA3, TM6SF2, and MBOAT7, further modulate susceptibility. Additionally, sex-specific factors influence disease development, with men and postmenopausal women showing higher prevalence.

4. Pathophysiology of MAFLD

The pathogenesis of MAFLD is multifactorial. While the original "two-hit" hypothesis emphasized the sequential roles of hepatic steatosis and oxidative injury, the current "multiple parallel hits" model better reflects the complexity of the disease. Factors including insulin resistance, dysbiosis of the gut microbiome, adipokine imbalance, and oxidative stress [1] interact simultaneously, leading to hepatic injury.

Lipid accumulation in hepatocytes sensitizes the liver to secondary insults such as ROS and inflammatory mediators. Mitochondrial dysfunction [2] plays a central role in this process. It not only promotes excessive ROS generation but also impairs beta-oxidation, leading to lipid overload and endoplasmic reticulum (ER) stress. Additionally, dysfunction in mitochondrial complexes disrupts ATP production, further exacerbating hepatocyte vulnerability.

5. Role of oxidative stress in MAFLD progression

Oxidative stress is defined as an imbalance between pro-oxidant and antioxidant forces in favor of the former. In MAFLD, this imbalance arises from increased ROS production and/or reduced antioxidant defenses. Mitochondria are the primary source of ROS through electron leakage from the electron transport chain (ETC). Enzymes such as NADPH oxidases and cytochrome P450s also contribute to ROS accumulation.

The consequences of oxidative stress [1] in MAFLD are multifaceted:

- Lipid peroxidation: ROS oxidize polyunsaturated fatty acids in cellular membranes, forming reactive aldehydes like malondialdehyde (MDA) and 4-hydroxynonenal (4-HNE), which further damage proteins and DNA.

- DNA damage: Oxidative stress [1] leads to mutations in mitochondrial and nuclear DNA, compromising cellular repair mechanisms.
- Protein oxidation: ROS induce post-translational modifications in key metabolic and structural proteins, impairing their function.

These effects collectively promote hepatocyte apoptosis [9], necrosis, and activation of fibrogenic pathways [6, 8–10].

6. Mitochondrial dysfunction and oxidative stress

Mitochondria are central to the pathophysiology of MAFLD. Dysfunctional mitochondria fail to efficiently metabolize fatty acids, resulting in lipid accumulation and increased ROS production. Pyruvate dehydrogenase (PDH) and α-ketoglutarate dehydrogenase (KGDH) are key mitochondrial enzymes involved in energy metabolism and are significant sources of ROS when impaired.

Studies show that PDH and KGDH generate mitochondrial hydrogen peroxide (mH2O2) under metabolic stress, contributing to both oxidative eustress (adaptive) and oxidative distress (pathologic) signaling. Furthermore, these enzymes are subject to redox [12] regulation *via* glutathionylation and nitrosylation, altering their activity in response to the cellular redox [12] environment (**Figure 2**).

7. Immune system involvement in oxidative stress

Oxidative stress also influences the hepatic immune microenvironment. Pattern recognition receptors (PRRs), such as Toll-like receptors (TLRs) and NOD-like

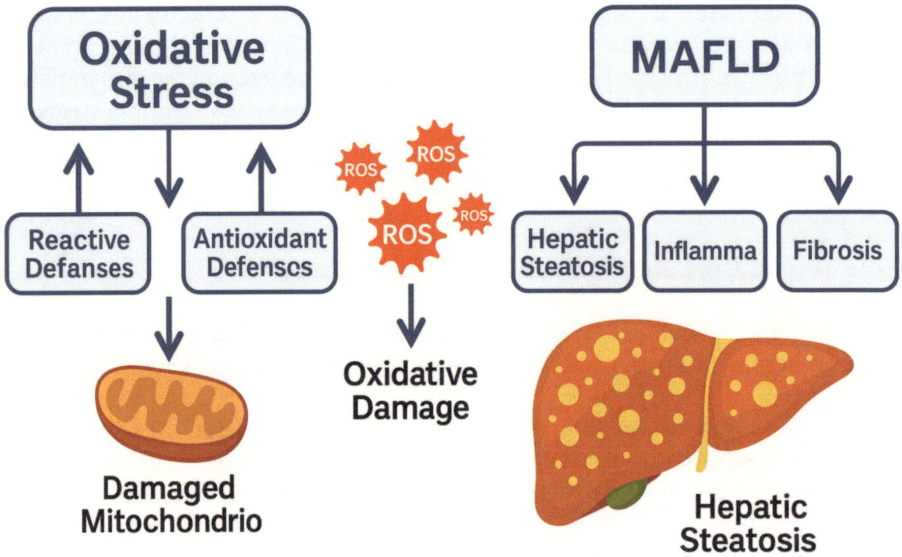

Figure 2.
Oxidative stress and mitochondrial damage.

receptors (NLRs), detect oxidative damage-associated molecules. Activation of NLRP3 inflammasome by ROS triggers the release of interleukins IL-1β and IL-18 *via* caspase-1, promoting liver inflammation [3].

Kupffer cells and recruited monocyte-derived macrophages amplify this inflammatory milieu, leading to hepatocyte death and fibrogenesis. Hepatic stellate cells (HSCs) are activated in response to ROS and cytokines, initiating extracellular matrix (ECM) deposition and fibrosis [8]. Chronic activation of these pathways contributes to NASH and cirrhosis [12–17].

8. Genetic and epigenetic modulators

Genetic predispositions significantly influence MAFLD susceptibility. Variants such as PNPLA3 I148M, TM6SF2 E167K, and MBOAT7 rs641738 are linked to disease progression and severity. These genes affect lipid metabolism, inflammation [3], and mitochondrial function.

Epigenetic mechanisms, including DNA methylation, histone modifications, and non-coding RNAs (e.g., miRNAs and lncRNAs), regulate gene expression in response to oxidative stress [1]. Notably, Nrf2, a transcription factor governing antioxidant responses, is epigenetically regulated and serves as a protective factor in MAFLD.

9. Antioxidant defense mechanisms

The body deploys enzymatic and non-enzymatic antioxidants [4] to counter ROS. Key antioxidant enzymes include:

- Superoxide dismutase (SOD): converts superoxide anions into hydrogen peroxide.
- Catalase (CAT): decomposes hydrogen peroxide into water and oxygen.
- Glutathione peroxidase (GPx): reduces peroxides using glutathione (GSH) [18].

Non-enzymatic antioxidants [4] include vitamin E, vitamin C, and GSH.
In MAFLD, these defense systems are often overwhelmed or downregulated, highlighting the potential role for therapeutic supplementation [19–27].

10. Diagnostic biomarkers of oxidative stress

Biomarkers such as MDA, 4-HNE, F2-isoprostanes, and advanced oxidation protein products (AOPPs) serve as indicators of oxidative damage. Antioxidant enzyme activities (SOD, CAT, GPx) and levels of GSH provide insights into redox [12] status. Imaging modalities and liver biopsies remain the gold standard for assessing fibrosis [8] but integrating oxidative markers can enhance diagnostic precision [20–25].

11. Therapeutic interventions targeting oxidative stress

Several antioxidants [4] have been explored for MAFLD treatment:

- Vitamin E (α-tocopherol): shown to reduce liver inflammation [3] and steatosis in clinical trials, neutralizes lipid radicals, inhibits peroxidation, and reduces inflammation and showed significant histological improvement in NASH patients. The PIVENS trial demonstrated that vitamin E (800 IU/day) significantly improved steatosis, inflammation, and hepatocellular ballooning in non-diabetic NASH patients compared to placebo [28]. However, concerns remain regarding its long-term safety, including potential associations with increased all-cause mortality and prostate cancer risk.

- N-acetylcysteine (NAC): precursor to glutathione; reduces transaminases and oxidative stress., with potential hepatoprotective effects.

- Polyphenols (e.g., resveratrol [15], curcumin [16]): natural compounds with antioxidant and anti-inflammatory properties, shown to reduce oxidative stress and inflammation in animal and pilot human studies.

- Mitochondria-targeted therapies: Compounds like MitoQ aim to restore mitochondrial function and reduce ROS production.

- Emerging therapies focus on modulating redox [12]-sensitive signaling pathways, including Nrf2 activation and inhibition of ROS-generating enzymes like NOX.

- Silymarin—antioxidant and antifibrotic effects *via* ROS scavenging and TGF-β inhibition.

- Other therapies—PPAR agonists (e.g., pioglitazone)—improve IR and reduce oxidative stress.

12. Lifestyle and dietary modifications

Lifestyle interventions are fundamental in MAFLD management. Weight loss through diet and exercise improves insulin sensitivity and reduces hepatic fat content. Diets rich in antioxidants [4, 19] (e.g., Mediterranean diet) and physical activity enhance endogenous antioxidant capacity and mitochondrial function.

Avoiding alcohol, processed foods, and high-fructose diets also mitigates oxidative stress [1]. Nutritional counseling and behavioral support increase adherence and efficacy.

13. Future directions and research gaps

Despite advances in understanding the pathophysiological role of oxidative stress in MAFLD, several gaps remain. It is still unclear whether oxidative stress is a primary trigger or a secondary consequence of metabolic dysregulation. Additionally, individual variability in antioxidant response, influenced by genetics and environmental factors, may explain the heterogeneous progression of MAFLD among patients. Therefore, future research should focus on identifying reliable biomarkers of oxidative stress and personalized treatment approaches based on oxidative profiles.

Despite growing knowledge, several questions remain:

- What are the long-term effects of antioxidant therapies?
- Can oxidative stress [1] biomarkers predict disease progression?
- How do redox [12, 19, 27] modifications influence gene expression and metabolism?

Addressing these questions requires longitudinal studies and integration of omics technologies (genomics, transcriptomics, metabolomics) to unravel the complex interplay between oxidative stress [1] and MAFLD.

14. The gut-liver axis and oxidative stress

The interplay between the gut microbiota [10] and the liver—known as the gut-liver axis—is increasingly recognized in the pathogenesis of MAFLD. Increased intestinal permeability, often seen in obesity and MAFLD, allows the translocation of bacterial endotoxins like lipopolysaccharide (LPS) into the portal circulation. ROS-induced damage to intestinal tight junctions exacerbates this permeability. LPS activates toll-like receptor 4 (TLR4) on Kupffer cells and hepatocytes, promoting further ROS production and inflammation, which exacerbates hepatic injury and promotes fibrogenesis. This feedback loop sustains liver injury and may accelerate disease progression.

Short-chain fatty acids (SCFAs), bile acids, and microbial metabolites such as trimethylamine N-oxide (TMAO) further modulate redox [12] balance and immune responses. Therapeutic strategies targeting the microbiota, including probiotics, prebiotics, and fecal microbiota transplantation, hold promise in modulating oxidative stress [1] and MAFLD progression.

15. Environmental and lifestyle exposures

In addition to pharmacological approaches, lifestyle interventions play a crucial role in reducing oxidative stress. Weight loss through calorie restriction and physical activity improves insulin sensitivity, reduces hepatic fat, and lowers markers of oxidative stress. Diets rich in antioxidants, such as the Mediterranean diet, have been associated with improved liver function and reduced MAFLD prevalence [29]. Regular physical activity enhances mitochondrial biogenesis and increases endogenous antioxidant capacity, providing long-term protection against oxidative damage.

Environmental pollutants, endocrine-disrupting chemicals (EDCs), and occupational toxins are emerging contributors to MAFLD through their role in oxidative stress [1] induction. Persistent organic pollutants such as dioxins and polychlorinated biphenyls (PCBs) can accumulate in adipose tissue and trigger mitochondrial dysfunction [2], leading to increased ROS production.

Sedentary behavior, chronic stress, and inadequate sleep also influence redox [12] homeostasis. These lifestyle factors upregulate cortisol and other stress-related mediators, which impair mitochondrial function and downregulate antioxidant defenses. Understanding these extrinsic risk factors is crucial for comprehensive prevention strategies (**Figure 3**) [27, 30–33].

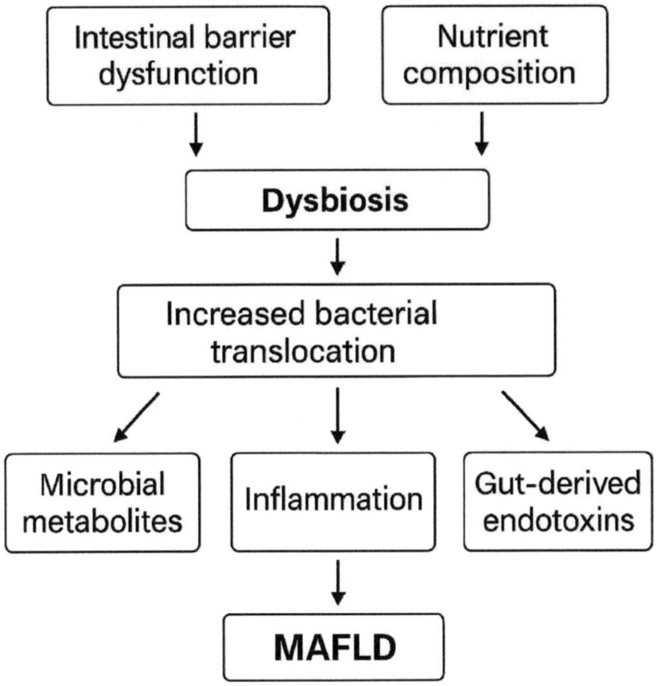

Figure 3.
Relation between nutrients, dysbiosis, and MAFLD.

16. Pediatric and adolescent MAFLD

MAFLD is not restricted to adults. Pediatric cases are rising in parallel with childhood obesity. In younger individuals, the disease often presents with more severe histological features, including periportal inflammation [3] and advanced fibrosis [8]. Oxidative stress [1] plays a similar mechanistic role in pediatric MAFLD, but the developing liver and immune system may respond differently to metabolic insults.

Antioxidant defenses in children may be less mature, rendering them more vulnerable to oxidative injury. Early-life exposures, including diet and environmental toxins, may have long-term epigenetic effects that predispose individuals to MAFLD later in life. This underscores the need for early screening and age-appropriate interventions.

17. Systems biology and multi-omics approaches

Systems biology and multi-omics technologies (genomics, transcriptomics, proteomics, and metabolomics) offer unprecedented insight into the complexity of MAFLD. These tools allow for the integration of vast datasets to identify novel biomarkers and therapeutic targets linked to oxidative stress [1].

For example, metabolomic profiling can reveal oxidative metabolites and disrupted redox [12] pathways, while transcriptomic data can uncover oxidative stress [1]-responsive gene networks. Machine learning models trained on omics datasets may predict disease progression and treatment response, paving the way for precision hepatology.

18. Conclusion

Oxidative stress [1] is a central mechanism in MAFLD pathogenesis, mediating hepatocyte injury, inflammation [3], and fibrosis [8]. mitochondrial dysfunction [2] and impaired antioxidant defenses exacerbate disease progression.

Oxidative stress mediates the harmful effects of metabolic overload by promoting lipid peroxidation, mitochondrial dysfunction, inflammation, and fibrogenesis. By impairing insulin signaling and altering the gut-liver axis, oxidative stress exacerbates the metabolic and immune disturbances characteristic of MAFLD.

Understanding these processes offers opportunities for early diagnosis and targeted interventions. Future research should aim to personalize treatments based on oxidative stress [1] profiles, enabling precision medicine approaches for MAFLD [34, 35]. While antioxidant therapies hold promise, they must be integrated into broader lifestyle and metabolic management strategies. A deeper understanding of oxidative pathways in MAFLD may pave the way for innovative, targeted interventions that could significantly reduce the burden of fatty liver disease worldwide.

Conflict of interest

The authors declare no conflict of interest.

Author details

Oana Timofte*, Alexandru Sidencu, Lilia Lica and Elena Gologan
"Grigore T Popa" University of Medicine and Pharmacy, Iasi, Romania

*Address all correspondence to: oanatimo@yahoo.com

References

[1] Clare K, Dillon JF, Brennan PN. Reactive oxygen species and oxidative stress in the pathogenesis of MAFLD. Journal of Clinical and Translational Hepatology. 2022;**10**(5):939-946. DOI: 10.14218/JCTH.2022.00067

[2] Hu Z, Yue H, Jiang N, Qiao L. Diet, oxidative stress and MAFLD: A mini review. Frontiers in Nutrition. 2025;**12**:1539578. DOI: 10.3389/fnut.2025.1539578

[3] Angelico F et al. Review and expert opinion on MAFLD, oxidative stress and multifunctional management. Drugs in Context. 2024;**13**:2023-2029. DOI: 10.7573/dic.2023-9-3

[4] Rani V et al. Oxidative stress and metabolic disorders: Pathogenesis and therapeutic strategies. Life Sciences. 2016;**148**:183-193. DOI: 10.1016/j.lfs.2016.02.002

[5] Li S et al. The role of oxidative stress and antioxidants in liver diseases. International Journal of Molecular Sciences. 2015;**16**:26087-260124. DOI: 10.3390/ijms161125942

[6] Cichoż-Lach H, Michalak A. Oxidative stress as a crucial factor in liver diseases. World Journal of Gastroenterology. 2014;**20**(25):8082-8091. DOI: 10.3748/wjg.v20.i25.8082

[7] Pastori D et al. Similar reduction of cholesterol-adjusted vitamin E serum levels in simple steatosis and non-alcoholic Steatohepatitis. Clinical and Translational Gastroenterology. 2015;**6**(10):e113. DOI: 10.1038/ctg.2015.43

[8] Seidita A et al. Oxidative stress as a target for non-pharmacological intervention in MAFLD: Could there be a role for EVOO? Antioxidants. 2024;**13**(6):731. DOI: 10.3390/antiox13060731

[9] Delli Bovi AP et al. Oxidative stress in non-alcoholic fatty liver disease. An updated mini review. Frontiers in Medicine. 2021;**8**:595371. DOI: 10.3389/fmed.2021.595371

[10] Zhang L et al. Biochemical basis and metabolic interplay of redox regulation. Redox Biology. 2019;**26**:101284. DOI: 10.1016/ j.redox.2019.101284

[11] He F et al. Redox mechanism of reactive oxygen species in exercise. Frontiers in Physiology. 2016;**7**:486. DOI: 10.3389/fphys.2016. 00486

[12] Klotz LO, Steinbrenner H. Cellular adaptation to xenobiotics: Interplay between xenosensors, reactive oxygen species and FOXO transcription factors. Redox Biology. 2017;**13**:646-654. DOI: 10.1016/j.redox.2017.07.015

[13] Wu D, Cederbaum AI. Alcohol, oxidative stress, and free radical damage. Alcohol Research & Health. 2003;**27**:277-284

[14] Jitcă G et al. Positive aspects of oxidative stress at different levels of the human body: A review. Antioxidants. 2022;**11**(3):572. DOI: 10.3390/antiox11030572

[15] Bardaweel SK et al. Reactive oxygen species: The dual role in physiological and pathological conditions of the human body. The Eurasian Journal of Medicine. 2018;**50**(3):193-201. DOI: 10.5152/eurasianjmed.2018.17397

[16] Tavassolifar MJ et al. The influence of reactive oxygen species in the

immune system and pathogenesis of multiple sclerosis. Autoimmune Diseases. 2020;**2020**:5793817. DOI: 10.1155/2020/5793817

[17] Chen Z et al. Role of oxidative stress in the pathogenesis of nonalcoholic fatty liver disease. Free Radical Biology & Medicine. 2020;**152**:116-141. DOI: 10.1016/j.freeradbiomed.2020.02.025

[18] Crosas-Molist E et al. Role of NADPH oxidases in the redox biology of liver fibrosis. Redox Biology. 2015;**6**:106-111. DOI: 10.1016/j.redox.2015.07.005

[19] Presa N et al. Vitamin E alleviates non-alcoholic fatty liver disease in phosphatidylethanolamine N-methyltransferase deficient mice. Biochimica et Biophysica Acta. 2019;**1865**:14-25. DOI: 10.1016/j.bbadis.2018.10.010

[20] Kisseleva T, Brenner DA. Role of hepatic stellate cells in fibrogenesis and the reversal of fibrosis. Journal of Gastroenterology and Hepatology. 2007;**22**(Suppl.1):S73-S78. DOI: 10.1111/j.1440-1746.2006.04658.x

[21] Ma Y et al. Oxidative stress is a key modulator in the development of nonalcoholic fatty liver disease. Antioxidants. 2022;**11**(1):91. DOI: 10.3390/antiox11010091

[22] Rolo AP et al. Role of oxidative stress in the pathogenesis of nonalcoholic steatohepatitis. Free Radical Biology & Medicine. 2012;**52**:59-69. DOI: 10.1016/j.freeradbiomed.2011.10.003

[23] Fang YL et al. Pathogenesis of non-alcoholic fatty liver disease in children and adolescence: From "two hit theory" to "multiple hit model". World Journal of Gastroenterology. 2018;**24**(27):2974-2983. DOI: 10.3748/wjg.v24.i27.2974

[24] Sugimoto H et al. Deletion of nuclear factor-E2-related factor-2 leads to rapid onset and progression of nutritional steatohepatitis in mice. American Journal of Physiology-Gastrointestinal and Liver Physiology. 2010;**298**:G283-G294. DOI: 10.1152/ajpgi.00296.2009

[25] Couto N et al. The role of glutathione reductase and related enzymes on cellular redox homoeostasis network. Free Radical Biology & Medicine. 2016;**95**:27-42. DOI: 10.1016/j.freeradbiomed.2016.02.028

[26] Swiderska M et al. Oxidative stress biomarkers in the serum and plasma of patients with non-alcoholic fatty liver disease (NAFLD). Can plasma AGE be a marker of NAFLD? Oxidative stress biomarkers in NAFLD patients. Free Radical Research. 2019;**53**:841-850. DOI: 10.1080/10715762.2019.1635691

[27] Martín-Fernández M et al. Role of oxidative stress and lipid peroxidation in the pathophysiology of NAFLD. Antioxidants. 2022;**11**(11):2217. DOI: 10.3390/antiox11112217

[28] Baratta F, Pastori D, Polimeni L, Bucci T, et al. Adherence to Mediterranean diet and non-alcoholic fatty liver disease: A systematic review and meta-analysis. Liver International. 2020;**40**(6):1327-1338. DOI: 10.1111/liv.14472

[29] Sanyal AJ, Chalasani N, Kowdley KV, et al. Pioglitazone, vitamin E, or placebo for nonalcoholic steatohepatitis. The New England Journal of Medicine. 2010;**362**(18):1675-1685

[30] Eslam M et al. A new definition for metabolic dysfunction-associated fatty liver disease: An international expert consensus statement. Journal of Hepatology. 2020;**73**:202-209. DOI: 10.1016/j.jhep. 2020. 03.039

[31] Eslam M et al. MAFLD: A consensus-driven proposed nomenclature for metabolic associated fatty liver disease. Gastroenterology. 2020;**158**:1999-2014.e1. DOI: 10.1053/j.gastro.2019.11.312

[32] Valenti LVC, Moretti V. Implications of the evolving knowledge of the genetic architecture of MASLD. Nature Reviews Gastroenterology & Hepatology. 2024;**21**(1):5-6. DOI: 10.1038/s41575-023-00866-0

[33] Mezzacappa C. Validation and epidemiologic definition of the novel steatotic liver disease nomenclature in a National United States cohort with cirrhosis. Clinical Gastroenterology and Hepatology. 2024;**15**:S1542-3565(24)01089-9. DOI: 10.1016/j.cgh.2024.10.035

[34] Feng Y et al. Protocatechuic acid relieves ferroptosis in hepatic lipotoxicity and steatosis via regulating NRF2 signaling pathway. Cell Biology and Toxicology. 2024;**40**:104. DOI: 10.1007/s10565-024-09953-7

[35] Huby T, Gautier EL. Immune cell-mediated features of non-alcoholic steatohepatitis. Nature Reviews Immunology. 2022;**22**:429-443. DOI: 10.1038/s41577-021-00639-3

Chapter 3

Perspective Chapter: From Plate to Pathophysiology – How Dietary Fats Drive Steatosis?

Fatemeh Maleki Sedgi and Borna AliBabazadeh

Abstract

Steatosis, the excessive accumulation of fat within liver cells, represents an early and reversible stage of liver disease that can progress to more severe conditions such as non-alcoholic fatty liver disease (NAFLD) and non-alcoholic steatohepatitis (NASH). Dietary fats play a pivotal role in the development and progression of hepatic steatosis through complex metabolic and molecular pathways. This chapter explores how different types of dietary fatty acids, including saturated, monounsaturated, and polyunsaturated fats, influence liver fat accumulation by modulating key processes such as *de novo* lipogenesis, fatty acid oxidation, and lipid storage. It further highlights the interplay between dietary fats, gut microbiota, and genetic predispositions that contribute to individual variability in steatosis susceptibility. The chapter also discusses the impact of lipotoxicity, mitochondrial dysfunction, and inflammatory signaling as critical drivers in the transition from simple steatosis to progressive liver injury. Finally, current nutritional strategies for prevention and treatment of steatosis are reviewed, emphasizing the importance of fat quality alongside overall dietary patterns. Understanding the molecular mechanisms linking dietary fats to steatosis offers promising avenues for personalized nutrition and therapeutic interventions aimed at halting the progression of liver disease at its earliest stage.

Keywords: steatosis, MAFLD, NAFLD, nutrition, diet, SFAs, PUFAs

1. Introduction

1.1 Overview of steatosis

The liver plays a pivotal role in maintaining homeostasis by regulating various physiological functions such as metabolism, detoxification, protein synthesis, and immune responses [1]. Liver diseases encompass a broad spectrum of conditions marked by hepatocellular injury, infiltration of inflammatory cells, and activation of hepatic stellate cells (HSCs), all of which contribute to impaired liver function and structural alterations [2]. Hepatic steatosis refers to the abnormal accumulation of triglycerides within hepatocytes. This condition primarily manifests in two major forms: non-alcoholic fatty liver disease (NAFLD) and alcoholic fatty liver disease (AFLD). However, several additional etiologies including metabolic disorders, nutritional imbalances, certain medications (such as chemotherapy agents and corticosteroids), and hepatitis C virus (HCV) infection also play a role in its development [2].

NAFLD is characterized by excessive lipid deposition in liver tissue, which may result from a variety of interrelated mechanisms. These include elevated lipolysis in adipose tissue or increased dietary fat consumption, both of which elevate circulating free fatty acids (FFAs) [3]. Mitochondrial dysfunction, commonly associated with insulin resistance a condition that often precedes NAFLD, can lead to impaired β-oxidation of fatty acids, further promoting lipid accumulation [3]. Additionally, enhanced *de novo* lipogenesis in the liver significantly contributes to hepatic fat storage [4]. Finally, a reduction in lipid clearance, frequently observed in individuals with insulin resistance, can further aggravate hepatic steatosis [5].

1.2 Epidemiology of steatosis

Liver disease remains one of the leading causes of mortality worldwide. According to the Global Burden of Disease Study 2019, approximately 1.26 million deaths were attributed to cirrhosis and other chronic liver conditions, reflecting a 13% increase since 1990 [6]. Liver cancer, often the final stage in the progression of liver disease, was responsible for nearly 830,000 deaths in 2020, accounting for 8.3% of all cancer-related fatalities globally [7]. Moreover, viral hepatitis particularly hepatitis B virus (HBV) and hepatitis C virus (HCV) continues to result in approximately 1.3 million deaths each year [8]. Alcohol-associated liver disease (ALD) also contributes significantly to the global burden, with an estimated 3.3 million new cases annually, accounting for roughly 5.9% of worldwide deaths [9]. In parallel, the mortality rate due to metabolic dysfunction-associated steatotic liver disease (MASLD) is rising, with around 280,000 deaths reported in 2019 [10]. Recent meta-analyses have identified MASLD as the most prevalent form of chronic liver disease, affecting approximately 38% of the global adult population between 2016 and 2019 [11]. Additionally, the incidence of ALD is increasing in tandem with global trends in alcohol consumption.

2. Understanding steatosis

2.1 Classification based on etiology

Hepatic steatosis is categorized according to its underlying causes, including NAFLD, ALD, metabolic disorders such as obesity, insulin resistance, and dyslipidemia, as well as steatosis associated with viral infections particularly hepatitis C and drug-induced liver injury resulting from hepatotoxic medications or environmental exposures. Given the strong correlation between NAFLD and metabolic risk factors, including obesity, type 2 diabetes mellitus (T2DM), and elevated triglyceride levels, an updated term metabolic (dysfunction)-associated fatty liver disease (MAFLD) has been introduced. This revised nomenclature underscores the metabolic basis of the condition and seeks to enhance diagnostic clarity and clinical relevance.

2.2 Non-alcoholic vs. alcoholic fatty liver disease

NAFLD is the most prevalent form of hepatic steatosis, affecting approximately 30–40% of men and 15–20% of women in the general population [12]. It is widely recognized as the hepatic manifestation of metabolic syndrome and is strongly associated with insulin resistance, atherosclerosis, obesity, dyslipidemia, and hypertension. The excessive accumulation of lipids within hepatocytes triggers oxidative stress and inflammatory pathways, potentially leading to non-alcoholic steatohepatitis (NASH), which may subsequently progress to liver fibrosis and cirrhosis [13]. NAFLD is projected to become the leading indication for liver transplantation by 2030. Another major etiology of hepatic steatosis is chronic alcohol consumption; AFLD is observed in up to 90% of individuals with alcohol use disorder [14]. Among those with isolated AFLD, approximately 10% are at risk of developing cirrhosis. Daily ethanol intake of 30 grams or more has been shown to significantly elevate the risk of chronic liver injury and cirrhosis. Moreover, factors such as female sex, cigarette smoking, obesity, and coexisting hepatic conditions further increase susceptibility to liver damage in individuals with AFLD.

2.3 Pathological stages

The pathological progression of steatosis, particularly within the framework of NAFLD, represents a continuum of hepatic damage. NAFLD serves as a broad classification encompassing a range of liver conditions, typically extending from simple steatosis (fat accumulation in the liver) to NASH, advancing further to steatohepatitis with fibrosis, and ultimately cirrhosis. Importantly, NAFLD leads to liver injury and fibrosis in the absence of alternative causes such as drug-induced liver damage, viral hepatitis, or excessive alcohol intake.

3. Dietary fats: Compositions and sources

3.1 Saturated fats

Dietary fat constitutes a vital nutrient and an integral component of every human cell. Rather than advocating for the elimination of dietary fat, it is crucial to comprehend the distinct roles of various fat types and their contributions to a balanced diet. Recent research identifies red meat and high-fat dairy products such as beef, butter, whole milk, cheese, and ice cream as the primary sources of saturated fatty acids (SFAs) [15]. Specifically, short- and medium-chain saturated fats predominantly derive from dairy products, whereas long-chain saturated fats are mainly present in red meat and high-fat dairy [15].

Fatty acids differ structurally, and their chemical configurations influence metabolic processing within the human body. Saturated fats, characterized by the absence of double bonds, consist of straight, densely packed molecules that solidify at room temperature [15]. Public health authorities, including the American Heart Association and the National Cholesterol Education Program, consistently recommend reducing intake of SFA and trans fatty acids (TFA) [16–18]. One practical approach to fulfilling these guidelines is to decrease the consumption of oils rich in SFAs. Moreover, *in vitro* studies across various cell types have demonstrated that excessive exposure to SFAs triggers the upregulation of pro-inflammatory cytokines, disrupts insulin signaling pathways, and induces apoptosis, accompanied by endoplasmic reticulum dysfunction and oxidative stress (**Table 1**) [19].

Type of fat	Chemical structure	Main dietary sources	Physiological/health effects
Saturated fatty acids (SFA)	No double bonds; straight chains, solid at room temperature	Red meat (beef), high-fat dairy (butter, whole milk, cheese, and ice cream)	Promotes inflammation, insulin resistance, ER stress, and oxidative stress; public health guidelines recommend reducing intake
Trans fatty acids (TFA)	Unsaturated with trans double bonds (mostly industrial origin)	Margarine, snack foods, baked goods, fried fast foods, and shortening	Linked to cardiovascular disease and metabolic disorders, industrial TFAs are widely restricted
Monounsaturated fatty acids (MUFA)	One double bond; bent structure, liquid at room temperature	Olive oil, avocado, nuts, some red meats, and dairy products	Generally beneficial; associated with improved lipid profiles and reduced liver fat
Polyunsaturated fatty acids (PUFA)	Multiple double bonds; highly flexible, remains liquid at lower temps	Soybean, corn, fish, flaxseed, vegetable oils	ω-6 (LA → AA) is pro-inflammatory; ω-3 (ALA → EPA, DHA) is anti-inflammatory and supports liver health
Cholesterol	Sterol ring structure, found in animal tissues	Eggs, shrimp, beef, poultry, cheese, butter	Essential for membranes and hormone synthesis; excessive intake linked to cardiovascular risk

Table 1.
Dietary fats: Composition, sources, and physiological effects.

3.2 Trans fats

TFAs are a type of unsaturated fatty acid that occur infrequently in natural sources but have been widely produced industrially since the 1950s through the partial hydrogenation of vegetable oils [20]. These industrially derived TFAs are commonly found in products such as margarines, snack foods, packaged baked goods, and fried items [21]. Epidemiological studies have consistently linked TFA consumption to an elevated risk of cardiovascular diseases and metabolic disorders [22]. However, further research is needed to elucidate the direct molecular mechanisms by which TFAs contribute to lipid abnormalities and hepatic steatosis. Although naturally occurring TFAs are present in minimal quantities in animal-derived foods such as meat and dairy, significant amounts are detected in processed items including shortening, bread, margarine, cream cakes, fried fast foods, and other industrially processed products [23]. The food industry frequently utilizes partially hydrogenated vegetable oils to improve the shelf life and sensory qualities of food products, which inadvertently leads to the formation of TFAs (**Table 1**).

3.3 MUFAs and PUFAs

Unsaturated fats are typically liquid at room temperature due to the presence of double bonds, which create structural kinks that prevent tight molecular packing. Monounsaturated fatty acids (MUFAs) contain a single double bond, introducing a bend in the fatty acid chain that results in fats that remain liquid at room temperature but solidify when chilled, as observed in oils such as olive and avocado oil. Polyunsaturated fatty acids (PUFAs), which possess multiple double bonds, are found in sources such as soybean, corn, fish, flaxseed, and most vegetable oils [15]. These multiple kinks maintain their liquid state even at lower temperatures by further inhibiting close packing of the molecules.

PUFAs are further classified based on the position of their double bonds, which influences their oxidation properties and metabolic pathways. Among PUFAs, the essential fatty acids α-linolenic acid (ALA; ω-3) and linoleic acid (LA; ω-6) have been extensively studied in relation to the progression of NAFLD. LA is metabolized into arachidonic acid (AA; 20:4 n-6), whereas ALA is converted into eicosapentaenoic acid (EPA; 20:5 n-3) and docosahexaenoic acid (DHA; 22:6 n-3). The metabolic derivatives of AA exert pro-inflammatory, pro-thrombotic, and pro-aggregatory effects. Conversely, EPA and DHA contribute to modulating hepatic lipid composition by enhancing anti-inflammatory mediators and reducing insulin resistance [24]. Notably, diminished hepatic levels of EPA and DHA may favor lipid synthesis (lipogenesis) over fatty acid β-oxidation, thereby promoting steatosis. Consequently, the ω-6 to ω-3 fatty acid ratio is critical in influencing the prevalence of chronic metabolic diseases, with imbalances particularly excessive ω-6 intake being implicated. Nonetheless, evidence from a double-blind randomized trial indicates that a long-term hypercaloric diet rich in ω-6 PUFAs may prevent hepatic fat accumulation in overweight individuals [25].

Dietary MUFAs primarily consist of oleic acid (cis-9-octadecenoic acid, comprising over 90%) and minor components such as palmitoleic acid (cis-9-hexadecenoic acid). Collectively, MUFAs contribute approximately 12% of total energy intake in the United States [26]. These fatty acids are derived from diverse sources, including plant-based foods (e.g., vegetable oils and nuts) and animal-based products (e.g., red meats and high-fat dairy), which exhibit varying health effects (**Table 1**) [27].

3.4 Dietary cholesterols

Cholesterol, a predominant sterol found in animal tissues, performs vital physiological functions in the human body. It serves as a fundamental structural component of cell membranes, contributing significantly to membrane fluidity. Additionally, cholesterol plays a critical role in the formation of lipid rafts, which are essential for processes such as protein sorting, cellular signaling, and apoptosis. Dietary cholesterol primarily originates from animal-derived foods, with key sources including egg yolks, shrimp, beef, pork, poultry, cheese, and butter. Data from the National Health and Nutrition Examination Survey (NHANES) 2005–2006 identified eggs and egg-based dishes, chicken, beef and beef-based dishes, burgers, and regular cheese as the top five contributors to cholesterol intake in the American population [28]. The hepatic cholesterol pool is maintained by two primary sources: exogenous cholesterol obtained from the diet and endogenous cholesterol synthesized *de novo* in the liver and extrahepatic tissues (**Table 1**) [29].

4. Mechanisms: How dietary fats influence hepatic fat accumulation?

Alterations in the levels of diverse lipid species, arising from an imbalance among lipolysis, lipid uptake, lipogenesis, and lipid oxidation or secretion, can lead to organelle dysfunction, including endoplasmic reticulum (ER) stress and mitochondrial impairment (**Table 2**).

4.1 Lipid metabolism (lipolysis) and hepatic lipid overload

The majority of patients with NAFLD exhibit increased white adipose tissue (WAT) mass, and the expansion of this tissue constitutes a significant risk factor in

Mechanism	Key processes	Main findings	Implications
1. Lipid metabolism and lipolysis	• Enhanced lipolysis in WAT • Redistribution from subcutaneous to visceral fat • Increased FFA flux to liver	• 60–70% of liver fat in NAFLD may derive from adipose lipolysis • Linked to inflammation and insulin resistance	• Visceral fat and dysregulated lipolysis are major contributors to hepatic fat overload
2. *De novo* lipogenesis (DNL)	• Conversion of carbs to fatty acids • Triggered by insulin resistance and high carb (esp. fructose) intake	• DNL accounts for ~20–30% of hepatic fat • Promotes TG synthesis and harmful lipid intermediates	• High carbohydrate diets, especially with fructose, worsen hepatic steatosis
3. Mitochondrial dysfunction and oxidative stress	• Impaired β-oxidation • Excess ROS production • Mitochondrial DNA damage	• SFAs (e.g., palmitic acid) disrupt mitochondrial function • Triggers inflammation, cell death	• Mitochondrial impairment links SFA intake with NASH progression
4. Gut microbiota alterations	• SFA intake reduces microbial diversity • PUFA has minimal effect • Stearic acid beneficial	• Microbiota changes mediate dietary fat effects on liver • Akkermansia increase linked with liver protection	• Microbiota modulation is a promising therapeutic target
5. Lipotoxicity	• Accumulation of toxic lipid species • ER stress, lysosomal damage, apoptotic signaling	• Ceramides, DAGs, and EVs drive inflammation and cell death	• Central to transition from simple steatosis to NASH

Table 2.
Summary of mechanisms linking dietary fats to hepatic steatosis and NAFLD progression.

NAFLD progression [30]. Clinical studies have demonstrated that a redistribution of fat storage from subcutaneous to visceral adipose depots correlates with hepatic injury, with visceral adipose tissue expansion serving as a strong predictor for NAFLD development [31]. However, further research is necessary to clarify the relationship between liver damage and alterations in the fatty acid composition within adipose tissue. As the principal source of circulating lipids, elevated free fatty acid (FFA) release from adipose tissue is closely linked to enhanced lipolysis, particularly increased triglyceride (TG) hydrolysis [32]. In obese NAFLD patients, augmented adipose tissue lipolysis may account for approximately 60–70% of hepatic fat accumulation [3]. This excessive lipolysis is also associated with dysregulated secretion of adipocyte-derived hormones, such as reduced adiponectin levels, and adipose tissue inflammation marked by the release of pro-inflammatory cytokines, both of which contribute to insulin resistance and thereby exacerbate ectopic lipid deposition [33].

Beyond cytosolic lipolysis, lipophagy a selective form of macroautophagy represents an alternative mechanism for TG hydrolysis [32]. Lipophagy facilitates the breakdown of triglycerides stored in lipid droplets through their sequestration and subsequent fusion with lysosomes. Notably, lipophagy plays a more prominent role in triglyceride catabolism within brown adipose tissue and the liver compared to WAT [34]. In NAFLD patients, chronic lipid overload is associated with impaired lipophagy, whereas acute lipid exposure *in vitro* has been shown to stimulate lipophagy, potentially reflecting an adaptive cellular response. Additionally, circulating FFAs originate not only from adipose tissue but also from the efflux of lipids from other cell types, including hepatocytes, as well as from triglyceride-rich lipoproteins hydrolyzed by lipoprotein lipase (LPL) [32].

4.2 Insulin resistance and *de novo* lipogenesis

De novo lipogenesis (DNL) is a cellular metabolic pathway that synthesizes fatty acids from acetyl-CoA and malonyl-CoA. Multiple clinical studies have reported an increased rate of DNL in obese patients with NAFLD, accounting for approximately 20–30% of hepatic fat accumulation [3, 35]. Mechanistically, elevated DNL is closely linked to insulin resistance (IR) and excessive carbohydrate consumption. IR impairs glucose oxidation and redirects carbohydrates toward the DNL pathway [36]. Notably, fructose exerts a more pronounced effect than glucose in stimulating DNL and triglyceride (TG) synthesis [37]. The upregulation of DNL occurs alongside enhanced *de novo* glycerolipid synthesis and subsequent TG accumulation, whereby FFAs are esterified into TG and stored in lipid droplets.

Beyond promoting TG synthesis, glycerolipid metabolism is a critical source of various lipid second messengers, including phosphatidic acid, lysophosphatidic acid, diacylglycerol (DAG), and other intermediates such as ceramides and sphingolipids. These lipid species have been implicated in the disruption of insulin signaling pathways and exert cytotoxic effects [38]. Although several lipidomics studies have identified aberrant glycerolipid metabolism in NAFLD patients, the precise molecular mechanisms underpinning these alterations remain largely unresolved [32].

4.3 Mitochondrial dysfunction and oxidative stress

Increased hepatic fatty acid flux and uptake do not consistently result in marked changes in mitochondrial β-oxidation, mitochondrial dysfunction is a well-documented feature of NASH. Liver biopsies from NASH patients and rodent models of NAFLD reveal impaired mitochondrial respiratory chain activity accompanied by distinct ultrastructural abnormalities, including mitochondrial enlargement, altered cristae morphology, loss of characteristic dense mitochondrial granules, and epigenetic modifications of mitochondrial DNA [39, 40]. Substantial evidence indicates that certain fatty acids, such as SFAs and ceramides, exert deleterious effects on mitochondrial integrity and function. Exposure to palmitic acid, for example, initially increases mitochondrial oxygen consumption rates twofold and promotes excessive reactive oxygen species (ROS) generation. This oxidative stress leads to the modification of proteins and lipids and disrupts cellular signaling pathways, partly through phosphatase inactivation [41]. Furthermore, palmitic acid stimulates the release of mitochondrial DNA into the extracellular milieu and activates c-Jun N-terminal kinase (JNK) in a manner dependent on the mitochondrial protein Sab (Sh3bp5) [42]. Free fatty acids also indirectly contribute to mitochondrial damage by promoting lysosomal membrane permeabilization, which triggers the activation of pro-apoptotic Bcl-2 family members, resulting in mitochondrial membrane permeabilization and the initiation of apoptotic cell death [43].

4.4 Gut microbiota and lipids

The quantity of dietary SFA significantly influences both liver health and the composition of the gut microbiota in humans. Variations in dietary fatty acid profiles impact liver steatosis, hepatic metabolism, and alter gut microbial communities. Notably, changes in SFA intake exert a more pronounced effect on the gut microbiota compared to equivalent variations in MUFA or PUFA consumption. A systematic review has demonstrated that diets high in SFA reduce the diversity and richness of the human gut microbiota, whereas PUFA-rich diets have minimal effects, and findings regarding MUFA-rich diets remain inconsistent [44]. Dietary intervention studies further indicate that SFA intake elevates hepatic fat accumulation more than PUFA or MUFA consumption, although epidemiological data on dietary risk factors for steatosis remain limited [45, 46]. The observed associations between dietary lipid composition, gut microbiota structure, and liver fat accumulation suggest a potential mediating role of the microbiota in lipid-induced steatosis [47]. *In vitro* studies have revealed that n-3 PUFAs regulate the activity of various transcription factors and suppress fatty acid synthesis in hepatocytes, with serum levels of n-3 PUFAs correlating with hepatic gene expression [48, 49]. Contrary to other long-chain SFAs, stearic acid has been associated with a favorable metabolic profile, including reductions in plasma cholesterol and hepatic fat deposition [50, 51]. Furthermore, stearic acid has recently been shown to mitigate liver injury and promote shifts in the gut microbiota, notably increasing *Akkermansia muciniphila* abundance in a murine model of alcoholic liver disease [52]. These findings highlight the therapeutic potential of modulating the gut microbiota through dietary lipids to influence liver steatosis.

4.5 Mechanisms of lipotoxicity

Lipotoxicity, characterized by lipid-induced cellular toxicity resulting in organelle dysfunction, aberrant activation of intracellular signaling pathways, chronic inflammation, and ultimately cell death, is a central feature of NASH [38, 53, 54]. The underlying mechanisms of lipotoxicity encompass multiple cellular processes, including ER stress, mitochondrial impairment, and lysosomal membrane permeabilization, which collectively culminate in cell death *via* apoptosis, necroptosis, or pyroptosis. Recent studies have highlighted that lipotoxicity can trigger the release of extracellular vesicles (EVs) and is intricately linked to hypoxic conditions, both of which contribute significantly to NAFLD progression. The subsequent sections summarize the latest advances in understanding the molecular and cellular pathways mediating lipotoxicity in NAFLD [32].

5. Evidence from studies

A growing body of evidence from both animal and human studies has elucidated the complex relationship between dietary lipids, gut microbiota, and hepatic steatosis. Schoeler et al. examined the effects of dietary fats on gut microbiota composition and liver steatosis in male mice [47]. Their findings indicated that poorly absorbed long-chain SFA, especially stearic acid, modified bile acid profiles and improved metabolic outcomes and liver fat accumulation. Notably, these effects occurred independently of dietary fiber intake, suggesting a direct interaction between certain SFAs and the gut-liver axis.

Similarly, research by Wit et al. demonstrated that diets high in saturated fats contribute to obesity and hepatic steatosis by altering gut microbiota through the increased delivery of dietary fats to the distal intestine [55]. The study revealed a strong inverse correlation between serum PUFA and liver fat content, while serum SFA levels showed a positive association with hepatic fat accumulation. In support of these findings, other studies have reported that individuals with NASH exhibit higher levels of SFA and lower levels of PUFA in liver triacylglycerols, with a clear trend of decreasing PUFA content corresponding to increasing NAFLD severity [56].

Further evidence from Sobrecases et al. indicated that a hypercaloric diet rich in SFA (comprising 30% of total energy intake, with 18% as SFA) resulted in a more significant increase in liver fat content (~86%) than a diet high in fructose (~16%) [57].

Human dietary intervention trials have reinforced these observations. Rosqvist et al. conducted a double-blind, randomized controlled trial in which lean individuals were overfed muffins enriched with either palm oil (SFA) or sunflower oil (PUFA), contributing approximately 750 additional kilocalories per day [58]. Despite equivalent weight gain across both groups, SFA intake led to greater fat accumulation in the liver and visceral adipose tissue, whereas PUFA intake was associated with an increase in lean body mass. Another study showed that overconsumption of SFA led to more than a 50% increase in hepatic fat, along with elevated ALT and ceramide levels. In contrast, PUFA overfeeding had no adverse effects on hepatic lipid levels and even slightly reduced liver fat while improving lipid profiles [25].

Consistent with these findings, Luukkonen et al. reported that 3 weeks of SFA overfeeding (+1000 kcal/day) in overweight men resulted in a 55% increase in liver fat, compared to 15 and 33% increases with unsaturated fatty acids (UFA) and simple sugars, respectively [59, 60]. Additionally, SFA intake was associated with a significant rise in insulin resistance.

Moreover, multiple human studies have highlighted the hepatoprotective effects of MUFA. Diets high in MUFA, even when isocaloric, have been shown to reduce hepatic fat content, particularly in individuals with NAFLD [60]. For example, Maleki Sedgi et al. found that substituting ghee with rapeseed oil rich in MUFA and PUFA resulted in significant improvements in liver steatosis, liver enzyme levels, glycemic control, and anthropometric parameters among patients with NAFLD [61].

6. Nutritional strategies for prevention and treatment

Due to the rising prevalence of NAFLD and its close links to numerous comorbidities and increased mortality, it is crucial that patients begin managing the condition immediately upon diagnosis. Currently, there are no approved medications specifically targeting NAFLD, although over 25 drugs are currently in phase 2 or 3 clinical trials [62]. As a result, treatment mainly focuses on weight loss and improving insulin resistance, achieved through lifestyle changes, medication, or endoscopic and surgical methods.

More than 16 randomized controlled trials have investigated the effects of weight loss through lifestyle modification on NAFLD [63]. Most of these studies have employed similar dietary strategies, aiming for either a daily caloric deficit between 300 and 1000 kcal or establishing a total daily calorie goal between 1200 and 1800 kcal, or 20–30 kcal per kilogram of body weight [63]. Many of these interventions also incorporate moderate-intensity physical activity, typically three to four sessions per week lasting 30–60 minutes each. These combined interventions have been compared to either standard care, minimal lifestyle advice, or exercise alone. A recent meta-analysis reported an average weight loss of around 3.6 kg from such programs. However, achieving resolution of more advanced liver disease, such as NASH, may require substantially greater weight reduction.

One prospective study followed nearly 300 patients with biopsy-confirmed NASH who were encouraged to lose weight through lifestyle changes and underwent liver biopsies at baseline and after 52 weeks [64]. The study found that the degree of weight loss was independently associated with improvements in liver histology related to NASH. While many interventions focus on well-balanced calorie restriction, certain dietary patterns might offer additional benefits, particularly those that enhance insulin sensitivity, which aligns with the underlying mechanisms of NAFLD.

Among the diets evaluated, the Mediterranean diet has received notable attention. This diet, characterized by high intakes of monounsaturated fats and omega-3 fatty acids, while limiting red meat, processed foods, and refined sugars, has shown promising effects. In a study involving obese patients with diabetes, those following the Mediterranean diet experienced the most significant decreases in liver enzyme levels, specifically ALT [65]. Importantly, these benefits persisted even after adjusting for potential confounders such as changes in body mass index, waist-to-hip ratio, and insulin resistance (**Figure 1**).

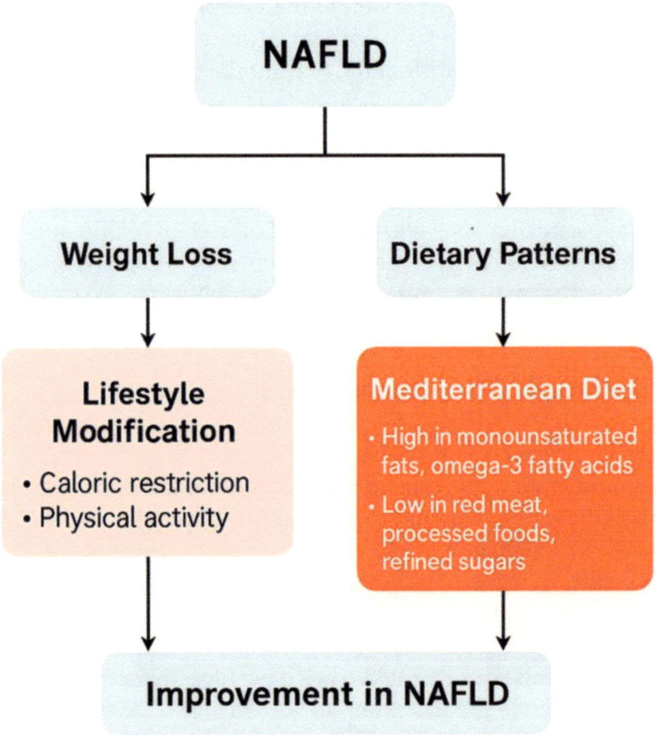

Figure 1.
Summary of nutritional management of NAFLD.

7. Future directions

As the global burden of continues to rise, alongside the growing awareness of the impact of dietary fats, future research must aim to uncover the precise molecular mechanisms through which different types of dietary fats influence liver fat accumulation and disease progression. While it is clear that saturated fats, trans fats, and imbalanced omega-6 to omega-3 ratios contribute to inflammation, oxidative stress, and insulin resistance, key drivers of NAFLD, there remains a critical need for more long-term human studies and rigorously controlled clinical trials to establish causality and deepen our understanding.

Additionally, exploring how genetic factors interact with gut microbiota and dietary fat metabolism could shed light on why some individuals are more susceptible to NAFLD and why responses to dietary interventions vary widely. Advanced omics approaches, including lipidomics, metabolomics, and transcriptomics, hold great promise for identifying new biomarkers and therapeutic targets that can differentiate between simple steatosis and its more severe, progressive forms like non-alcoholic steatohepatitis (NASH).

Another promising but underexplored area is the influence of dietary fats on autophagy processes, particularly lipophagy the selective degradation of lipid droplets. Understanding how certain fats modulate lipophagy could open new avenues for restoring healthy lipid metabolism in the liver and preventing disease advancement.

Finally, these scientific insights should inform public health policies and nutritional guidelines, moving beyond a focus on fat quantity alone to emphasize fat quality and overall dietary patterns. Such guidelines should also consider lifestyle factors to provide a holistic approach to preventing and managing NAFLD, reflecting the nuanced roles of different fat types in liver health.

8. Conclusion

Current dietary guidelines often overlook individual differences in metabolism and genetics that shape responses to diet, highlighting the value of personalized nutrition. While reducing saturated fat intake is recommended, its exact effects on liver health remain complex and may vary by fat source and genetic background. Diets high in saturated fats can increase liver fat and oxidative stress, whereas unsaturated fats may help protect the liver. The role of trans fats is still unclear due to limited human research. Overall, considering both fat type and individual variability could improve strategies for preventing and managing NAFLD.

Acknowledgements

The authors would like to express their sincere gratitude to the Maternal and Childhood Obesity Research Center, Urmia University of Medical Sciences, for their support and provision of research resources. We are also grateful to the Department of Biology, Faculty of Sciences, Urmia University, for their academic guidance and encouragement throughout the development of this chapter.

Fatemeh Maleki Sedgi was responsible for the supervision, conceptualization, investigation, original drafting of the manuscript, and preparation of visual materials. Borna AliBabazadeh contributed to critical review and editing of the manuscript, validation of scientific content, and methodological support. Both authors reviewed and approved the final version of the manuscript.

Conflict of interest

The authors declare no conflict of interest.

Author details

Fatemeh Maleki Sedgi[1*] and Borna AliBabazadeh[2]

1 Maternal and Childhood Obesity Research Center, Urmia University of Medical Sciences, Urmia, Iran

2 Faculty of Sciences, Department of Biology, Urmia University, Urmia, Iran

*Address all correspondence to: f.maleki1998@gmail.com

References

[1] Santos AA, Delgado TC, Marques V, Ramirez-Moncayo C, Alonso C, Vidal-Puig A, et al. Spatial metabolomics and its application in the liver. Hepatology. 2024;**79**(5):1158-1179

[2] Angulo P. Obesity and nonalcoholic fatty liver disease. Nutrition Reviews. 2007;**65**(suppl_1):S57-S63

[3] Donnelly KL, Smith CI, Schwarzenberg SJ, Jessurun J, Boldt MD, Parks EJ. Sources of fatty acids stored in liver and secreted via lipoproteins in patients with nonalcoholic fatty liver disease. The Journal of Clinical Investigation. 2005;**115**(5):1343-1351

[4] Postic C, Girard J. Contribution of de novo fatty acid synthesis to hepatic steatosis and insulin resistance: Lessons from genetically engineered mice. The Journal of Clinical Investigation. 2008;**118**(3):829-838

[5] Fabbrini E, Mohammed BS, Magkos F, Korenblat KM, Patterson BW, Klein S. Alterations in adipose tissue and hepatic lipid kinetics in obese men and women with nonalcoholic fatty liver disease. Gastroenterology. 2008;**134**(2):424-431

[6] Sepanlou SG, Safiri S, Bisignano C, Ikuta KS, Merat S, Saberifiroozi M, et al. The global, regional, and national burden of cirrhosis by cause in 195 countries and territories, 1990-2017: A systematic analysis for the global burden of disease study 2017. The Lancet Gastroenterology & Hepatology. 2020;**5**(3):245-266

[7] Cao W, Qin K, Li F, Chen W. Comparative study of cancer profiles between 2020 and 2022 using global cancer statistics (GLOBOCAN). Journal of the National Cancer Center. 2024;**4**(2):128-134

[8] Stanaway JD, Flaxman AD, Naghavi M, Fitzmaurice C, Vos T, Abubakar I, et al. The global burden of viral hepatitis from 1990 to 2013: Findings from the global burden of disease study 2013. The Lancet. 2016;**388**(10049):1081-1088

[9] Rehm J, Taylor B, Mohapatra S, Irving H, Baliunas D, Patra J, et al. Alcohol as a risk factor for liver cirrhosis: A systematic review and meta-analysis. Drug and Alcohol Review. 2010;**29**(4):437-445

[10] Le MH, Yeo YH, Li X, Li J, Zou B, Wu Y, et al. 2019 global NAFLD prevalence: A systematic review and meta-analysis. Clinical Gastroenterology and Hepatology. 2022;**20**(12):2809-17. e28

[11] Wong VW-S, Ekstedt M, Wong GL-H, Hagström H. Changing epidemiology, global trends and implications for outcomes of NAFLD. Journal of Hepatology. 2023;**79**(3):842-852

[12] Browning JD, Szczepaniak LS, Dobbins R, Nuremberg P, Horton JD, Cohen JC, et al. Prevalence of hepatic steatosis in an urban population in the United States: Impact of ethnicity. Hepatology. 2004;**40**(6):1387-1395

[13] Idilman IS, Ozdeniz I, Karcaaltincaba M. Hepatic steatosis: Etiology, patterns, and quantification. In: Seminars in Ultrasound, CT and MRI. Philadelphia, PA: Elsevier; 2016

[14] Mandayam S, Jamal MM, Morgan TR. Epidemiology of alcoholic liver disease. In: Seminars in Liver Disease. New York, NY: Thieme Medical Publishers, Inc.; 2004

[15] Gershuni VM. Saturated fat: Part of a healthy diet. Current Nutrition Reports. 2018;**7**:85-96

[16] Grundy SM. Third report of the national cholesterol education program (NCEP) expert panel on detection, evaluation, and treatment of high blood cholesterol in adults (adult treatment panel III) final report. Circulation. 2002;**106**:3143-3421

[17] Lichtenstein AH, Appel LJ, Brands M, Carnethon M, Daniels S, Franch HA, et al. Diet and lifestyle recommendations revision 2006: A scientific statement from the American Heart Association nutrition committee. Circulation. 2006;**114**(1):82-96

[18] Johnson GH, Keast DR, Kris-Etherton PM. Dietary modeling shows that the substitution of canola oil for fats commonly used in the United States would increase compliance with dietary recommendations for fatty acids. Journal of the American Dietetic Association. 2007;**107**(10):1726-1734

[19] Hu FB, Stampfer MJ, Manson JE, Ascherio A, Colditz GA, Speizer FE, et al. Dietary saturated fats and their food sources in relation to the risk of coronary heart disease in women. The American Journal of Clinical Nutrition. 1999;**70**(6):1001-1008

[20] Kris-Etherton PM, Lefevre M, Mensink RP, Petersen B, Fleming J, Flickinger BD. Trans fatty acid intakes and food sources in the US population: NHANES 1999-2002. Lipids. 2012;**47**(10):931-940

[21] Mozaffarian D, Katan MB, Ascherio A, Stampfer MJ, Willett WC. Trans fatty acids and cardiovascular disease. New England Journal of Medicine. 2006;**354**(15):1601-1613

[22] Jacome-Sosa MM, Borthwick F, Mangat R, Uwiera R, Reaney MJ, Shen J, et al. Diets enriched in trans-11 vaccenic acid alleviate ectopic lipid accumulation in a rat model of NAFLD and metabolic syndrome. The Journal of Nutritional Biochemistry. 2014;**25**(7):692-701

[23] Sommerfeld M. Trans unsaturated fatty acids in natural products and processed foods. Progress in Lipid Research. 1983;**22**(3):221-233

[24] de Castro GS, Calder PC. Non-alcoholic fatty liver disease and its treatment with n-3 polyunsaturated fatty acids. Clinical Nutrition. 2018;**37**(1):37-55

[25] Rosqvist F, Kullberg J, Ståhlman M, Cedernaes J, Heurling K, Johansson H-E, et al. Overeating saturated fat promotes fatty liver and ceramides compared with polyunsaturated fat: A randomized trial. The Journal of Clinical Endocrinology & Metabolism. 2019;**104**(12):6207-6219

[26] Joris PJ, Mensink RP. Role of cis-monounsaturated fatty acids in the prevention of coronary heart disease. Current Atherosclerosis Reports. 2016;**18**:1-7

[27] Praagman J, Beulens JW, Alssema M, Zock PL, Wanders AJ, Sluijs I, et al. The association between dietary saturated fatty acids and ischemic heart disease depends on the type and source of fatty acid in the European prospective investigation into cancer and nutrition–Netherlands cohort. The American Journal of Clinical Nutrition. 2016;**103**(2):356-365

[28] Xu Z, McClure ST, Appel LJ. Dietary cholesterol intake and sources among US adults: Results from National Health and nutrition examination surveys (NHANES), 2001-2014. Nutrients. 2018;**10**(6):771

[29] Soliman GA. Dietary cholesterol and the lack of evidence in cardiovascular disease. Nutrients. 2018;**10**(6):780

[30] Bedossa P, Tordjman J, Aron-Wisnewsky J, Poitou C, Oppert J-M, Torcivia A, et al. Systematic review of bariatric surgery liver biopsies clarifies the natural history of liver disease in patients with severe obesity. Gut. 2017;**66**(9):1688-1696

[31] Cimini FA, Barchetta I, Ciccarelli G, Leonetti F, Silecchia G, Chiappetta C, et al. Adipose tissue remodelling in obese subjects is a determinant of presence and severity of fatty liver disease. Diabetes/Metabolism Research and Reviews. 2021;**37**(1):e3358

[32] Geng Y, Faber KN, de Meijer VE, Blokzijl H, Moshage H. How does hepatic lipid accumulation lead to lipotoxicity in non-alcoholic fatty liver disease? Hepatology International. 2021;**15**:21-35

[33] Khan RS, Bril F, Cusi K, Newsome PN. Modulation of insulin resistance in nonalcoholic fatty liver disease. Hepatology. 2019;**70**(2):711-724

[34] Zechner R, Madeo F, Kratky D. Cytosolic lipolysis and lipophagy: Two sides of the same coin. Nature Reviews Molecular Cell Biology. 2017;**18**(11):671-684

[35] Fabbrini E, Luecking CT, Love-Gregory L, Okunade AL, Yoshino M, Fraterrigo G, et al. Physiological mechanisms of weight gain– induced steatosis in people with obesity. Gastroenterology. 2016;**150**(1):79-81. e2

[36] Geisler CE, Renquist BJ. Hepatic lipid accumulation: Cause and consequence of dysregulated glucoregulatory hormones. The Journal of Endocrinology. 2017;**234**(1):R1-R21

[37] Jensen T, Abdelmalek MF, Sullivan S, Nadeau KJ, Green M, Roncal C, et al. Fructose and sugar: A major mediator of non-alcoholic fatty liver disease. Journal of Hepatology. 2018;**68**(5):1063-1075

[38] Musso G, Cassader M, Paschetta E, Gambino R. Bioactive lipid species and metabolic pathways in progression and resolution of nonalcoholic steatohepatitis. Gastroenterology. 2018;**155**(2):282-302. e8

[39] Pirola CJ, Gianotti TF, Burgueño AL, Rey-Funes M, Loidl CF, Mallardi P, et al. Epigenetic modification of liver mitochondrial DNA is associated with histological severity of nonalcoholic fatty liver disease. Gut. 2013;**62**(9):1356-1363

[40] Einer C, Hohenester S, Wimmer R, Wottke L, Artmann R, Schulz S, et al. Mitochondrial adaptation in steatotic mice. Mitochondrion. 2018;**40**:1-12

[41] Egnatchik RA, Leamy AK, Noguchi Y, Shiota M, Young JD. Palmitate-induced activation of mitochondrial metabolism promotes oxidative stress and apoptosis in H4IIEC3 rat hepatocytes. Metabolism. 2014;**63**(2):283-295

[42] Win S, Than TA, Zhang J, Oo C, Min RWM, Kaplowitz N. New insights into the role and mechanism of c-Jun-N-terminal kinase signaling in the pathobiology of liver diseases. Hepatology. 2018;**67**(5):2013-2024

[43] Li Z, Berk M, McIntyre TM, Gores GJ, Feldstein AE. The lysosomal-mitochondrial axis in free fatty acid–induced hepatic lipotoxicity. Hepatology. 2008;**47**(5):1495-1503

[44] Wolters M, Ahrens J, Romaní-Pérez M, Watkins C, Sanz Y, Benítez-Páez A, et al. Dietary fat, the gut microbiota, and metabolic health–a systematic review conducted within the MyNewGut project. Clinical Nutrition. 2019;**38**(6):2504-2520

[45] Yki-Järvinen H, Luukkonen PK, Hodson L, Moore JB. Dietary carbohydrates and fats in nonalcoholic fatty liver disease. Nature Reviews Gastroenterology & Hepatology. 2021;**18**(11):770-786

[46] Hydes T, Alam U, Cuthbertson DJ. The impact of macronutrient intake on non-alcoholic fatty liver disease (NAFLD): Too much fat, too much carbohydrate, or just too many calories? Frontiers in Nutrition. 2021;**8**:640557

[47] Schoeler M, Ellero-Simatos S, Birkner T, Mayneris-Perxachs J, Olsson L, Brolin H, et al. The interplay between dietary fatty acids and gut microbiota influences host metabolism and hepatic steatosis. Nature Communications. 2023;**14**(1):5329

[48] Botolin D, Wang Y, Christian B, Jump DB. Docosahexaneoic acid (22: 6, n-3) regulates rat hepatocyte SREBP-1 nuclear abundance by Erk-and 26S proteasome-dependent pathways. Journal of Lipid Research. 2006;**47**(1):181-192

[49] Pawar A, Jump DB. Unsaturated fatty acid regulation of peroxisome proliferator-activated receptor α activity in rat primary hepatoctes. Journal of Biological Chemistry. 2003;**278**(38):35931-35939

[50] Gouk S-W, Cheng S-F, Ong AS-H, Chuah C-H. Stearic acids at sn-1, 3 positions of TAG are more efficient at limiting fat deposition than palmitic and oleic acids in C57BL/6 mice. British Journal of Nutrition. 2014;**111**(7):1174-1180

[51] Hassel CA, Mensing EA, Gallaher DD. Dietary stearic acid reduces plasma and hepatic cholesterol concentrations without increasing bile acid excretion in cholesterol-fed hamsters. The Journal of Nutrition. 1997;**127**(6):1148-1155

[52] Nie W, Xu F, Zhou K, Yang X, Zhou H, Xu B. Stearic acid prevent alcohol-induced liver damage by regulating the gut microbiota. Food Research International. 2022;**155**:111095

[53] Liangpunsakul S, Chalasani N. Lipid mediators of liver injury in nonalcoholic fatty liver disease. American Journal of Physiology-Gastrointestinal and Liver Physiology. 2019;**316**(1):G75-G81

[54] Mota M, Banini BA, Cazanave SC, Sanyal AJ. Molecular mechanisms of lipotoxicity and glucotoxicity in nonalcoholic fatty liver disease. Metabolism. 2016;**65**(8):1049-1061

[55] De Wit N, Derrien M, Bosch-Vermeulen H, Oosterink E, Keshtkar S, Duval C, et al. Saturated fat stimulates obesity and hepatic steatosis and affects gut microbiota composition by an enhanced overflow of dietary fat to the distal intestine. American Journal of Physiology-Gastrointestinal and Liver Physiology. 2012;**303**(5):G589-GG99

[56] Kaikkonen JE, Würtz P, Suomela E, Lehtovirta M, Kangas AJ, Jula A, et al. Metabolic profiling of fatty liver in young and middle-aged adults: Cross-sectional and prospective analyses of the Young Finns study. Hepatology. 2017;**65**(2):491-500

[57] Sobrecases H, Lê K-A, Bortolotti M, Schneiter P, Ith M, Kreis R, et al. Effects of short-term overfeeding with fructose, fat and fructose plus fat on plasma and hepatic lipids in healthy men. Diabetes & Metabolism. 2010;**36**(3):244-246

[58] Rosqvist F, Iggman D, Kullberg J, Cedernaes J, Johansson H-E, Larsson A, et al. Overfeeding polyunsaturated and saturated fat causes distinct

effects on liver and visceral fat accumulation in humans. Diabetes. 2014;**63**(7):2356-2368

[59] Luukkonen PK, Sädevirta S, Zhou Y, Kayser B, Ali A, Ahonen L, et al. Saturated fat is more metabolically harmful for the human liver than unsaturated fat or simple sugars. Diabetes Care. 2018;**41**(8):1732-1739

[60] Hodson L, Rosqvist F, Parry SA. The influence of dietary fatty acids on liver fat content and metabolism. Proceedings of the Nutrition Society. 2020;**79**(1):30-41

[61] Sedgi FM, Hosseiniazar MM, Alizadeh M. The effects of replacing ghee with rapeseed oil on liver steatosis and enzymes, lipid profile, insulin resistance and anthropometric measurements in patients with non-alcoholic fatty liver disease: A randomised controlled clinical trial. British Journal of Nutrition. 2024;**131**(12):1985-1996

[62] Friedman SL, Neuschwander-Tetri BA, Rinella M, Sanyal AJ. Mechanisms of NAFLD development and therapeutic strategies. Nature Medicine. 2018;**24**(7):908-922

[63] Koutoukidis DA, Astbury NM, Tudor KE, Morris E, Henry JA, Noreik M, et al. Association of weight loss interventions with changes in biomarkers of nonalcoholic fatty liver disease: A systematic review and meta-analysis. JAMA Internal Medicine. 2019;**179**(9):1262-1271

[64] Vilar-Gomez E, Martinez-Perez Y, Calzadilla-Bertot L, Torres-Gonzalez A, Gra-Oramas B, Gonzalez-Fabian L, et al. Weight loss through lifestyle modification significantly reduces features of nonalcoholic steatohepatitis. Gastroenterology. 2015;**149**(2):367-78. e5

[65] Fraser A, Abel R, Lawlor D, Fraser D, Elhayany A. A modified Mediterranean diet is associated with the greatest reduction in alanine aminotransferase levels in obese type 2 diabetes patients: Results of a quasi-randomised controlled trial. Diabetologia. 2008;**51**:1616-1622

Section 2

Lifestyle and Medical Intervention in MAFLD

Chapter 4

Perspective Chapter: Lifestyle Interventions for Hepatic Steatosis – Cornerstone of Management in Metabolic Dysfunction-Associated Steatotic Liver Disease

Yaoxin Wu, Huiling Gao, Chang Liu and Shan Gao

Abstract

This chapter wang to explore the pivotal role of lifestyle interventions as the first-line therapeutic strategy for managing hepatic steatosis in metabolic dysfunction-associated steatotic liver disease (MASLD). It delves into evidence-based approaches to dietary optimization, physical activity regimens, and sustainable weight loss, emphasizing their direct impact on reducing liver fat, improving metabolic parameters, and halting disease progression. Key topics include macronutrient composition (e.g., Mediterranean diet (MD), low-carbohydrate approaches), exercise modalities (aerobic vs. resistance training), and behavioral strategies to enhance adherence. The chapter also addresses challenges in patient engagement, cultural considerations in lifestyle modification, and the integration of multidisciplinary care teams. Practical clinical tools, such as patient-centered goal-setting frameworks and monitoring protocols, are highlighted to empower healthcare providers in translating research into effective, individualized care plans.

Keywords: hepatic steatosis, MASLD, lifestyle interventions, dietary, exercise, patient adherence

1. Introduction

Metabolic dysfunction-associated steatotic liver disease (MASLD), formerly known as nonalcoholic fatty liver disease (NAFLD), is defined as a hepatic steatosis that occurs in the absence of excessive alcohol consumption or other known causes of liver injury, with the presence of at least one cardiometabolic risk factor [1, 2]. As the incidence rates of obesity and type 2 diabetes (T2D) continue to rise globally, the prevalence of metabolic dysfunction-associated steatotic liver disease (MASLD) is also increasing [3]. Currently, 38% of adults and 7–14% of children/adolescents are affected by MASLD. By 2040, the prevalence of MASLD in adults is projected to exceed 55%. The most common cause of mortality among MASLD patients remains cardiovascular disease. Beyond hepatic outcomes (e.g., cirrhosis and hepatocellular carcinoma [HCC]), MASLD is associated with an elevated risk of developing incident type 2 diabetes (T2D), chronic kidney disease, sarcopenia, and extrahepatic malignancies. Furthermore, MASLD correlates with diminished health-related quality of life (HRQoL), reduced work productivity, fatigue, increased healthcare resource utilization, and substantial economic burdens (**Figure 1**) [4].

The hallmark feature of MASLD is excessive hepatic lipid accumulation, which may progress to steatohepatitis and fibrosis, posing significant threats to human health and lifespan [5]. The primary risk factors for MASLD encompass obesity, insulin resistance, hypertension, and hypertriglyceridemia, while its diagnosis concurrently serves to confirm the presence of underlying metabolic risk factors [6]. Current research indicates that MASLD has a multifactorial pathogenesis. Hepatic steatosis triggers oxidative stress, organelle dysfunction, apoptosis, and other pathophysiological alterations, all of which drive disease progression from MASLD to metabolic dysfunction-associated steatohepatitis (MASH) and hepatic fibrosis [7]. As the central hub of lipid metabolism, the liver regulates lipid homeostasis through four primary pathways: (1) uptake of circulating lipids, (2) *de novo* lipogenesis (DNL), (3) fatty acid oxidation (FAO), and (4) lipid export *via* very-low-density lipoprotein (VLDL). These processes are modulated by intricate interactions among hormones, nuclear receptors, and transcription factors, with dysregulation of hepatic lipid homeostasis leading to MASLD development. Similar to other metabolic disorders, lifestyle interventions—such as adopting a healthy diet and increasing physical activity—remain the cornerstone of MASLD management [8]. While no specific therapeutic agents have been unequivocally established for MASLD to date, lifestyle interventions represent a direct and accessible modality. This approach aligns with the multifactorial etiology of metabolic diseases, as lifestyle modifications can simultaneously target multiple pathophysiological pathways contributing to disease progression.

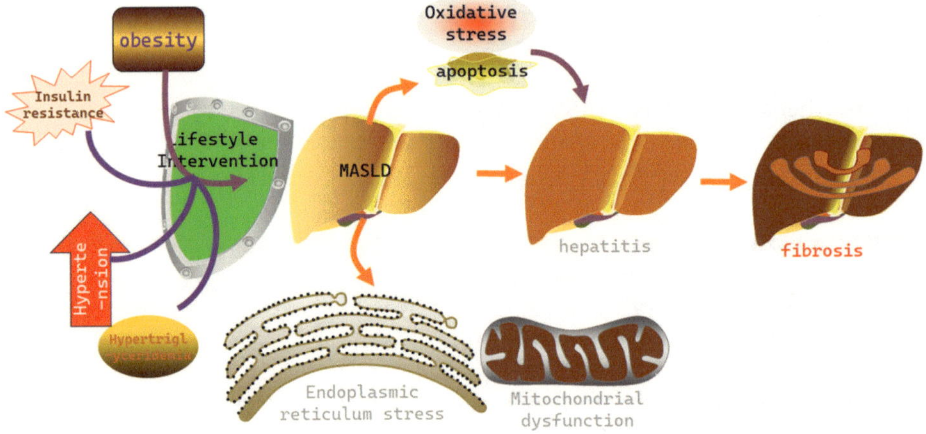

Figure 1.
The inducement and development of MASLD.

2. Relationship between MASLD and hepatic steatosis

It is well-established that the liver, as the central regulatory organ for lipid homeostasis, orchestrates four tightly regulated metabolic pathways: (1) *de novo* lipogenesis (DNL), (2) fatty acid uptake, (3) very-low-density lipoprotein (VLDL) secretion, and (4) fatty acid β-oxidation (FAO). These pathways collectively maintain a dynamic equilibrium of hepatic lipids [9]. Unhealthy lifestyles such as overeating and physical inactivity create a chronic energy surplus in the body. This disrupts the dynamic regulation of hepatic lipids, leading to excessive fat accumulation and the development of simple hepatic steatosis. Lipid overload in hepatocytes triggers mitochondrial dysfunction, endoplasmic reticulum (ER) stress, and NADPH oxidase activation, resulting in massive intracellular release of reactive oxygen species (ROS) and subsequent oxidative stress [10]. Under the dual assault of lipid metabolic dysregulation and oxidative stress, pattern recognition receptors (PRRs) in hepatocytes—such as nucleotide-binding oligomerization domain (NOD)-like receptors and Toll-like receptors (TLRs)—detect persistently generated pathogen-associated molecular patterns (PAMPs), damage-associated molecular patterns (DAMPs), and lipid metabolites. This activates downstream immune signaling pathways, including MAPK-JNK and NF-κB, ultimately inducing hepatocyte injury and hepatic inflammation. Additionally, when lipotoxicity-driven inflammation and hepatocyte damage occur, hepatic stellate cells (HSCs) are activated and transdifferentiate into proliferative, migratory, and contractile myofibroblasts. These cells enhance the transcription of fibrosis-related genes, secrete excessive collagen, and drive hepatic fibrogenesis [11]. Early-stage simple hepatic steatosis is clinically insidious, with minimal patient symptoms. Compounded by the current lack of effective therapeutic regimens and dynamic biomarkers, patients often miss the reversible therapeutic window. Approximately 20% of cases progress to metabolic dysfunction-associated steatohepatitis (MASH), with nearly 20% of MASH patients already exhibiting F2 fibrosis (≥stage 2) at diagnosis. Once progression reaches advanced stages, the disease may evolve into hepatocellular carcinoma (HCC) or even hepatic failure, leading to drastically reduced survival rates [12]. Impaired mitochondrial fatty acid oxidation (FAO) in hepatocytes leads to lipid accumulation, excessive reactive oxygen species (ROS) production, and oxidative damage, driving the pathogenesis of nonalcoholic fatty liver disease (NAFLD) [13]. Fatty acid translocase (cluster of differentiation 36 [CD36]), a transmembrane protein facilitating long-chain fatty acid (LCFA) uptake, has recently been linked to FAO. The functionality of CD36 is closely associated with its subcellular localization. Palmitoylation, one of the most common lipid modifications, regulates CD36 localization. Studies reveal CD36 localization on hepatocyte mitochondria. Palmitoylation of CD36 is significantly upregulated in NAFLD. Inhibition of CD36 palmitoylation markedly increases its mitochondrial distribution in hepatocytes. Depalmitoylated CD36 on mitochondrial membranes enhances FAO by promoting fatty acid transport into mitochondria. Mitochondria-enriched CD36 interacts with long-chain acyl-CoA synthetase 1 (ACSL1), thereby channeling more LCFAs to ACSL1. This increases long-chain acyl-CoA production, enhancing FAO and alleviating NAFLD [14].

Receptor-interacting protein kinase 3 (RIPK3) mediates NAFLD progression. Research demonstrates that RIPK3 deficiency ameliorates impairments in mitochondrial biogenesis, bioenergetics, and function in hepatocytes. RIPK3 deletion coincides with robust upregulation of antioxidant systems, reducing oxidative stress under lipid overload *in vivo* and *in vitro*. RIPK3-deficient hepatocytes exhibit smaller but more numerous lipid droplets (LDs) after free fatty acid exposure. RIPK3 deficiency upregulates LD-associated proteins perilipin 1 (PLIN1) and PLIN5 in adipocytes and the liver. PLIN1 overexpression modulates LD structure, mitigates mitochondrial stress during fatty acid overload, and correlates with reduced NAFLD severity in humans. Conversely, pathogenic PLIN1 frameshift variants are linked to NAFLD, fibrosis, and elevated hepatic RIPK3 levels in familial partial lipodystrophy [15].

Vacuole membrane protein 1 (VMP1), an endoplasmic reticulum (ER)-transmembrane protein, regulates autophagosome and lipid droplet formation [16]. Hepatocyte-specific deletion of VMP1 severely impairs very-low-density lipoprotein (VLDL) secretion, leading to massive hepatic steatosis, hepatocyte death, inflammation, and fibrosis—hallmarks of nonalcoholic steatohepatitis (NASH) [17]. Mechanistically, VMP1 deficiency reduces hepatic phosphatidylcholine (PC) and phosphatidylethanolamine (PE) levels and alters phospholipid composition. Experimental findings indicate that VMP1 deletion in the liver also causes neutral lipid accumulation within ER bilayers and impaired mitochondrial β-oxidation. Overexpression of VMP1 ameliorates diet-induced NASH by restoring VLDL secretion. These studies demonstrate that reduced hepatic VMP1 expression correlates with human NAFLD/NASH [16]. Forkhead box A3 (FOXA3), a member of the FOX family, plays a critical role in metabolic homeostasis. Under ER stress conditions, spliced X-box binding protein 1 (XBP1s) specifically induces FOXA3 transcription. FOXA3 exacerbates excessive lipid accumulation triggered by acute ER stressors like tunicamycin (TM), whereas hepatocyte-specific FOXA3 deficiency alleviates this phenotype. Notably, FOXA3 deletion reduces diet-induced chronic ER stress, hepatic steatosis, and insulin resistance. Moreover, FOXA3 inhibition *via* siRNA or adeno-associated virus (AAV) delivery improves fatty liver phenotypes. Mechanistically, FOXA3 directly regulates Period1 (Per1) transcription, which in turn promotes the expression of lipogenic genes, including SREBP1c, thereby enhancing lipid synthesis. Pathophysiologically, hepatic levels of FOXA3, Per1, and SREBP1c are elevated in obese individuals and NAFLD patients [18]. In addition to the conventional understanding that body fat originates from lipid-rich dietary sources, carbohydrates can be converted into fat through *de novo* lipogenesis (DNL)—a process upregulated in fatty liver disease. Biochemically, DNL involves the polymerization and reduction of acetyl-CoA, utilizing NADPH as an electron donor [19]. Studies employing stable isotope tracing demonstrate that adipose tissue DNL is supported by glucose and its catabolism *via* the pentose phosphate pathway to generate NADPH. In contrast, the liver derives acetyl-CoA for lipogenesis from acetate and lactate, while NADPH is sourced from folate-mediated serine catabolism. This NADPH production involves a cytosolic serine pathway in the liver, operating in the reverse direction compared to most tissues and tumors. Here, NADPH is generated through the SHMT1-MTHFD1-ALDH1L1 reaction sequence. Inhibition of serine hydroxymethyltransferase (SHMT) reduces hepatic lipogenesis, indicating that hepatic folate metabolism uniquely supports cytosolic NADPH production and fat synthesis. Critically, while the same enzymatic machinery drives lipogenesis in both liver and adipose tissues, these organs utilize distinct substrate sources. This divergence highlights potential therapeutic targets for intervention [20].

While the U.S. FDA has approved Resmetirom for treating adults with non-cirrhotic steatohepatitis and moderate-to-severe hepatic fibrosis (stages F2–F3), drug development for metabolic dysfunction-associated steatohepatitis (MASH) remains challenging. Although numerous pharmaceutical companies are pursuing MASH therapies, only a few agents—such as semaglutide and lanifibranor—have advanced smoothly into Phase 3 clinical trials. Metabolic surgery represents another therapeutic avenue for fatty liver disease; however, current evidence lacks high-quality, prospective, randomized controlled studies to validate its safety profile. Most existing studies have not reported postoperative adverse events. Consequently, lifestyle interventions combined with stratified management remain essential for MASLD management [21].

3. Dietary interventions and nutritional optimization

Emerging evidence indicates that dietary patterns in MASLD patients are associated with pro-inflammatory responses and increased risk of severe hepatic steatosis, characterized by excessive intake of added sugars, sugar-sweetened beverages, processed foods, and nonalcoholic baked goods [22]. Chronic high-fat diets (HFDs) induce excessive hepatic lipid deposition, leading to structural and functional liver abnormalities. HFD significantly alters the expression of Hedgehog (Hh) signaling pathway genes, particularly upregulating Sonic Hedgehog (Shh), Indian Hedgehog (Ihh), Hedgehog-interacting protein (Hhip), Patched1 (Ptch1), Smoothened (Smo), and *Glioma-associated oncogene homologs (Gli1/2/3)*. These changes correlate with histopathological features such as inflammatory cell infiltration, sinusoidal dilation, cellular necrosis, and microvesicular steatosis [23]. The hepatotoxic effects of HFD are primarily driven by a "two-hit" mechanism that exacerbates nonalcoholic fatty liver disease (NAFLD) progression: First Hit: Excessive lipid intake (particularly from Western-style diets) overwhelms hepatic metabolic capacity, causing aberrant lipid deposition. This process is tightly linked to insulin resistance, which not only enhances *de novo* lipogenesis (DNL) but also impairs fatty acid transport, aggravating hepatocyte steatosis [24]. Second Hit: Lipid overload triggers mitochondrial dysfunction, endoplasmic reticulum (ER) stress, and oxidative stress, disrupting hepatocyte metabolism and activating inflammatory cascades. These events drive the transition from simple steatosis to nonalcoholic steatohepatitis (NASH) [25]. Long-term HFD synergizes with obesity and dyslipidemia (components of metabolic syndrome) to amplify hepatic lipotoxicity, ultimately increasing risks of cirrhosis and hepatocellular carcinoma (HCC). Notably, even in nonobese individuals, HFD-induced dyslipidemia independently elevates NAFLD risk, underscoring the pivotal role of dietary modulation in liver health [26].

3.1 Clinical manifestations of MASLD caused by improper diet

In the early stage of MASLD, most patients have no obvious symptoms, and liver enzymes are usually found to be elevated by imaging examination (such as abdominal B-ultrasound) or blood examination during a health examination. The following mild symptoms may occur: ① Fatigue: the patient often feels tired and depressed; ② Right epigastric discomfort: slight swelling, pain, or oppression; ③ Dyspepsia: such as abdominal distension and belching. ④ Weight gain or obesity: especially abdominal obesity. When the disease develops to the middle stage, with the progress of the disease, the fatty degeneration of hepatocytes is aggravated, and the following manifestations may appear: ① Abnormal liver function: alanine aminotransferase (ALT) and Aspartate aminotransferase (AST) are increased; ② Insulin resistance: blood sugar rises after meals, and acanthosis nigricans appears on the skin (neck and armpit become black and thick); ③ Hyperlipidemia: the blood lipid (triglyceride, cholesterol) increased; ④ Metabolic syndrome: accompanied by hypertension, hyperglycemia, obesity, etc. If the dietary disharmony and metabolic problems persist for a long time, what is more serious is that MASLD can progress to metabolic steatohepatitis (MASH) and further develop into liver fibrosis, cirrhosis, and even liver cancer. It may be manifested as obvious fatigue, persistent pain in the right upper abdomen, dull complexion, itchy skin, jaundice (yellow skin and eyeball), ascites, edema of lower limbs, liver palms, and spider nevus.

3.2 Dietary recommendations

To effectively counteract the detrimental effects of carbohydrates in MASLD patients, the ketogenic diet (KD)—a novel low-carbohydrate dietary regimen—has been explored. Initially developed in the 1920s for clinical management of epilepsy, particularly in patients refractory to antiseizure medications [27], KD has garnered significant attention in recent decades for its beneficial roles in metabolic syndrome, neurological disorders, cardiovascular diseases, and cancer. The KD composition typically comprises 3–5% carbohydrates, 20–27% protein, and 70–75% lipids, inducing nutritional ketosis to shift energy metabolism toward fat breakdown. This metabolic state reduces blood glucose levels, enhances insulin sensitivity, and promotes weight loss in overweight/obese individuals [28]. In preclinical studies of HFD-induced MASLD, KD suppresses disease progression by modulating inflammatory pathways. Specifically, KD induces interleukin-6 (IL-6) production, which activates c-Jun N-terminal kinase (JNK). This cascade inhibits aberrant insulin signaling, thereby ameliorating hepatic steatosis and insulin resistance [29]. The Mediterranean diet (MD) is widely recognized for its emphasis on plant-based foods, supplemented by an appropriate amount of olive oil, healthy dairy products, and fish, which together provide patients with anti-inflammatory and antioxidant benefits [30]. In one study, patients followed two plant-based food/cautious diet strategies: the American Heart Association (AHA) diet (55% carbohydrate, 15% protein, 30% lipid) and the MD diet (40–45% carbohydrate, 25% protein, 30–35% lipid). The results showed that both of them could inhibit inflammatory markers, including leptin, adiponectin, M30, and LECT2. The Mediterranean diet (MD) prevents MASLD through various mechanisms. First of all, MD is rich in antioxidant and anti-inflammatory components, such as vitamin E, acids, and carotenoids, which help to reduce oxidative stress and inflammatory reactions, thus protecting the liver from damage. Oxidative stress is an important pathogenic mechanism of MASLD, and antioxidants such as vitamin E can effectively alleviate this process [31]. Secondly, MD's characteristics of low sugar, low fat, and high fiber are helpful in controlling weight and preventing obesity and diabetes. Unsaturated fatty acids in olive oil can improve insulin sensitivity and reduce cholesterol levels, thus promoting metabolic health. In addition, omega-3 fatty acids in fish can reduce inflammatory factors, promote fatty acid oxidation, and reduce liver fat accumulation [32]. MD can also improve intestinal health, promote intestinal peristalsis, maintain healthy intestinal microecology, and reduce the burden on the liver through rich dietary fiber. At the same time, folic acid and vitamins B6 and B12 in MD are helpful to improve cardiovascular health and reduce the risk of cardiovascular diseases [33]. Generally speaking, the Mediterranean diet has become an effective dietary pattern to prevent MASLD by regulating metabolism, reducing inflammatory reaction, protecting the liver, and improving overall health [34].

Next, taking the Mediterranean diet as an example, it introduces the recipe selection and the corresponding mechanism [35, 36].

1. The diet is rich in fruits, vegetables, and whole grains. The Mediterranean diet emphasizes the intake of rich, fresh fruits, vegetables, and whole grains. For example, tomatoes are rich in lycopene, which has a strong antioxidant effect and can inhibit cholesterol oxidation, thus reducing the risk of cardiovascular diseases [37]. Whole grains such as wheat, barley, oats, rice, highland barley, and corn are rich in dietary fiber, vitamins, and minerals, which help to maintain cardiovascular health. In the process of food processing and cooking, high temperatures and excessive processing should be minimized to avoid the loss of nutrients.

2. Olive oil is the core of the Mediterranean diet, and it is rich in monounsaturated fatty acids, especially oleic acid, which helps to reduce the level of low-density lipoprotein cholesterol (LDL-C) and maintain the level of high-density lipoprotein cholesterol (HDL-C) [38]. In addition, polyphenols in olive oil have antioxidant and anti-inflammatory effects, which can improve blood rheology and reduce thrombosis, thus reducing the risk of myocardial infarction and other cardiovascular events.

3. Nuts and beans are important sources of high-quality fat, vegetable protein, and soluble fiber. Beans have a low glycemic index, which can release blood sugar smoothly and reduce total cholesterol and triglyceride levels by increasing bile acid excretion and regulating liver lipid metabolism [39]. Eating about 25 grams of soy protein every day, combined with a diet with low cholesterol and saturated fat, can significantly reduce the risk of cardiovascular disease. At the same time, beans also have certain preventive and adjuvant therapeutic effects on some chronic diseases such as cancer, diabetes, and chronic kidney disease.

4. Spices cannot only enhance the flavor of food but also reduce the use of oil and salt in cooking and promote healthy eating habits. Many spices are rich in natural antioxidants, such as allicin and allicin, which have anti-inflammatory, antibacterial, blood pressure, and cholesterol-lowering effects [40]. Studies have shown that long-term consumption of garlic can reduce the risk of hypertension by more than one-third and improve blood viscosity, which has a positive impact on cardiovascular health.

5. Yogurt, cheese, and the Mediterranean diet advocate daily intake of fermented dairy products such as yogurt and cheese. This kind of food is rich in calcium, which is beneficial to bone health and especially suitable for middle-aged and elderly people. In addition, choosing low-fat or skim dairy products can reduce the intake of saturated fat and cardiovascular risk while obtaining nutrition.

6. Fish and seafood are the main sources of protein in the Mediterranean diet, especially deep-sea fish such as tuna, herring, sardine, salmon, and bream, which are rich in ω-3 polyunsaturated fatty acids (such as EPA and DHA). These fatty acids have multiple physiological functions, such as anti-inflammatory, antithrombotic, and heart rate regulation, which can significantly reduce the incidence of cardiovascular diseases [41]. In addition, omega-3 fatty acids can also prevent or alleviate depression, arthritis, and other diseases. When cooking fish, high-temperature frying should be avoided to preserve its nutritional value.

7. Red meat and eggs. It is suggested to limit the intake frequency and quantity of red meat (such as pork, beef, and mutton) in the Mediterranean diet and give priority to lean meat. Comparatively speaking, poultry meat is rich in protein and low in saturated fat, which is more beneficial to cardiovascular health. It is suggested to control the ratio of fat to lean when processing meat; for example, the content of lean meat in meat stuffing should reach above 90%. Eggs are an important source of high-quality protein, especially suitable for vegetarians or people who eat less meat.

8. Adequate water intake has a positive effect on the body's metabolic function and mental state. Although some studies suggest that moderate drinking of red wine may be beneficial to cardiovascular health, most patients are advised to avoid alcohol intake as much as possible.

However, special attention should be paid to patients with gastric ulcers and short bowel syndrome, who should reduce high-fiber food, and children, who need to increase their intake of high-quality protein. The choice of cooking methods should avoid frying and overprocessing and give priority to steaming, boiling, and cold salad.

4. Intervention in sports activities and its strategies

4.1 Mechanism of relieving MASLD by exercise

In addition to dietary intervention, physical exercise is also an effective strategy to treat nonalcoholic fatty liver disease (NAFLD). Exercise intervention can reduce the formation of lipid droplets and liver triglycerides induced by a high-fat diet. Exercise intervention enhances lipid intake by activating the AMPK/ULK1 pathway, respectively. In addition, exercise stimulates the production of FGF21 in muscle, which is then secreted into circulation and promotes lipid uptake in the liver through the AMPK-dependent pathway. It should be noted that fat accumulation will aggravate liver aging, which can be alleviated by exercise and diet intervention [42]. A study on the mechanism of exercise inhibiting the development of nonalcoholic fatty liver disease in mice induced by a high-fat diet (HFD) found that C57BL/6 J mice aged 6 weeks were fed a normal diet or HFD for 12 weeks and then induced to swim or stay sedentary for 8 weeks. NAFLD mice showed obvious steatosis, fibrosis, and liver injury, and the expressions of HMGCS2, Wnt3a/β-catenin, and phosphorylated (p)-AMPK in the liver increased. Exercise significantly reduced these symptoms and lowered the level of Wnt3a/β-catenin in lipotoxic liver tissue. The inhibition of HMGCS2 expression decreased the activation of the Wnt3a/β-catenin pathway and decreased the p-AMPK in HepG2 treated with palmitic acid. That is to say, exercise can prevent NAFLD-related liver injury, steatosis, and fibrosis. Exercise-mediated liver protection is partly achieved by blocking the upregulation of HMGCS2 and weakening the Wnt3a/β-catenin pathway [43]. It is found that swimming can reduce the lipid accumulation in the liver and improve the pathological changes of the liver. In addition, swimming reduced the excessive production of NOX4-derived reactive oxygen species (ROS) and reduced the level of formaldehyde (MDA). At the same time, swimming has an anti-apoptosis effect, which can decrease the expression of apoptosis-related genes (caspase 3, bax) by increasing the expression of anti-apoptosis factor bcl2. From the mechanism, the swimming intervention activated lipid metabolism and inflammation mediated by the SIRT1/AMPK signal and enhanced the activation of AKT and NRF2 and upregulated the downstream antioxidant genes [44].

However, exercise is not carried out alone, and it often needs to be carried out together with diet intervention. The research shows that compared with the control group, the weight, fat mass, waist circumference, and alanine aminotransferase (ALT) level of the participants in the diet-exercise joint experiment decreased significantly, while the insulin sensitivity increased significantly. Intermittent fasting combined with exercise can effectively reduce hepatic steatosis in patients with NAFLD, but it may not have additional benefits compared with fasting alone [45]. A study to test the combined effects of Time-Restricted Eating (TRE) and resistance exercise training (RT) on obesity and NAFLD in mice fed with a high-fat diet showed that TRF—8 of hours food intake—and RT—including stair climbing three times a week—reduced weight gain, improved blood sugar homeostasis, and reduced lipid accumulation in the liver. TRF combined with radiotherapy improved the respiratory exchange rate, energy consumption, and mitochondrial respiration of the liver. In addition, the analysis of gene expression in the liver showed that in the TRF + RT group, the mRNA expression of lipogenesis and inflammation genes was low, while the mRNA expression of fatty acid oxidation genes was increased. Importantly, TRF + RT has been proven to be more effective in preventing obesity and metabolic disorders. That is to say, compared with the single intervention, TRF and RT play a complementary role, which has a significant impact on the metabolic disorder and NAFLD in mice. When combined with RT, TRF provides additional benefits and is more effective than each intervention alone in increasing energy consumption, preventing weight gain, and regulating blood glucose homeostasis [46].

4.2 Lack of sports to promote the mechanism of MASLD

When there is a lack of physical exercise, the first thing that bears the brunt is excess energy, which in turn leads to fat deposition in the liver. If the dietary calorie intake is unchanged or increased, it will further make the calorie surplus, and the excess energy will accumulate in the liver cells in the form of triglycerides, which will lead to fatty degeneration of the liver and form MASLD. Exercise can improve the sensitivity of muscles to insulin, while lack of exercise can lead to increased insulin resistance, especially in skeletal muscle, adipose tissue, and liver. If insulin resistance occurs, it will lead to ① the increase of lipolysis, which leads to the release of free fatty acids (FFA) into the blood; ② the intake of FFA in the liver increases, and then the triglyceride synthesized in the liver increases; and ③ insulin resistance will also inhibit the output of liver fat, which will eventually show more and more liver fat. Lack of exercise will also lead to hypertrophy of adipose tissue and sustained release of inflammatory factors (such as TNF-α and IL-6), which will destroy the structure of liver cells, induce apoptosis and fibrosis of liver cells, and finally promote the development of MASLD steatohepatitis. Intestinal flora is also a link that cannot be ignored. Lack of exercise is related to the imbalance of intestinal flora. Healthy exercise can promote the growth of probiotics and maintain the intestinal barrier function. When intestinal permeability increases, endotoxin (LPS) may enter the blood, induce a hepatic inflammatory reaction, and aggravate hepatic steatosis. Exercise can strengthen the antioxidant enzyme system (such as SOD and GSH), while a lack of exercise will increase the level of oxidative stress in the body, damage the hepatocyte membrane, promote lipid peroxidation, and aggravate liver inflammation and fibrosis.

4.3 Suggested exercise mode

When adopting corresponding exercises, the first exercise is aerobic exercise and resistance exercise. Aerobic exercise can activate metabolism and liver fat consumption, including types of exercise like brisk walking, jogging, swimming, cycling, elliptical machine, and so on. Recommended five times a week, 30–45 minutes each time, moderate intensity (heart rate reaches 60–70% of the maximum heart rate, that is, "can talk but cannot sing"). Further, intermittent high-intensity interval training (HIIT) can be added, such as 30-second sprint +1-minute jogging alternately, twice a week. Aerobic exercise activates the AMPK pathway, enhances mitochondrial function, and accelerates fat decomposition and energy supply in the liver and muscle. Studies have shown that regular aerobic exercise can reduce liver fat content by 6–10% (which is independently related to weight loss). In addition, aerobic exercise increased the expression of the GLUT4 transporter in skeletal muscle, decreased the fasting insulin level, and inhibited the *de novo* synthesis of liver fat (DNL). It can also reduce pro-inflammatory factors (such as TNF-α and IL-6), upregulate antioxidant enzymes (SOD and glutathione), and reduce oxidative stress damage to the liver [47–49]. Resistance exercise can reconstruct muscle metabolism and protect the liver. Its forms include dumbbell/barbell training, elastic belt training, and self-weight training (squats, push-ups). It is recommended to do 8–10 movements 2–3 times a week, 8–12 times in each group (reaching 70–80% of exhaustion). And give priority to training large muscle groups (legs, back, chest), taking into account the core muscle groups (flat support). Resistance exercise stimulates muscle protein synthesis, improves basal metabolic rate (about 50–70 kcal per day for every 1 kg of muscle), and indirectly reduces liver fat accumulation. On the other hand, muscle, as a "metabolic buffer pool," can reduce the fluctuation of blood sugar and liver lipid regeneration by increasing glucose intake and glycogen storage. Studies have proved that resistance training can reduce the liver fat content of patients with MASLD by 5–8%. This may be achieved by promoting the release of muscle factors such as IL-15, inhibiting the inflammation of adipose tissue, and blocking the vicious circle of "liver-adipose tissue" [50, 51].

However, the combined effect of the two is better than that of a single exercise. Aerobic exercise directly consumes fat, while resistance exercise increases muscle metabolic capacity and improves insulin resistance and adiponectin levels together. However, the selection of different groups of people should be adjusted accordingly. For example, obese MASLD patients should mainly take low-impact aerobic exercise (swimming and cycling) in the early stage to avoid joint injury and gradually join resistance training with weight loss. The elderly or sarcopenia patients should focus on low-intensity resistance (elastic belt, sitting training) and balance training (Tai Chi) to prevent falls and maintain muscle function. People with diabetes need to pay attention to avoid fasting exercise and monitor blood sugar before and after exercise; resistance training is arranged 1 hour after meals to reduce the risk of hypoglycemia. During the exercise intervention, attention should be paid to gradual progress. At the same time, liver function (ALT, GGT), liver fat content (controlled attenuation parameter (CAP) value), and body composition (muscle/fat ratio) should be detected every three months. If the liver cirrhosis is decompensated, high-intensity exercise should be avoided, and training should be suspended in acute hepatitis.

5. Weight management and psychological intervention

5.1 Weight management

Obesity is a complex chronic disease and a global public health challenge. Obesity is characterized by excessive accumulation of body fat, which greatly increases the risk of many diseases, including nonalcoholic fatty liver disease, and is related to shortened life expectancy. Although lifestyle intervention (diet and exercise) has a significant effect on weight management, it is extremely challenging to achieve long-term successful weight loss, and the prevalence of obesity continues to rise around the world. In the past decades, the pathophysiology of obesity has been widely studied, and more and more signal transduction pathways are related to obesity, which makes it possible to fight obesity in a more effective and accurate way [52]. It is found that the same percentage of weight loss can be achieved at slow or fast speed (range: 0.2–3.2 kg/week) through dietary calorie restriction, exercise, and weight loss surgery. Compared with the slow weight loss rate, the faster weight loss rate may lead to more fat-free mass and less fat mass loss in the dynamic stage of weight loss and, at the same time, reduce the resting energy consumption to a greater extent. However, after 2–4 weeks of stabilization at a new low weight, these differences are weakened, and the rate and amount of weight recovery after 9–33 months are not affected (nor does it affect the tissue composition of weight recovery). Waist circumference, visceral fat and liver fat content, resting blood pressure, fasting blood lipid profile, insulin, and fat factor concentration show little difference under different weight loss rates. After rapid weight loss of 6–11%, the decrease of fasting blood glucose concentration and the improvement of insulin sensitivity are greater than those after gradual weight loss, but there is no difference after weight loss of 18–20%. After losing the same weight at different rates, the changes in body composition and metabolism are similar to a great extent, and occasional differences may have no clinical significance for the long-term management of obesity and cardiac metabolic diseases [53]. The research shows that compared with the control group, exercise training subjects are more likely to achieve a relative reduction of liver fat measured by MRI of ≥30% (odds ratio 3.51, 95% confidence interval 1.49–8.23, P = 0.004). A task of minutes/week with an exercise dose of ≥750 metabolic equivalents (for example, a brisk walk of 150 minutes/week) leads to a significant therapeutic response (MRI response odds ratio is 3.73, 95% confidence interval is 1.34–10.41, P = 0.010), but a small dose of exercise does not. Treatment response is independent of clinically significant weight loss (> 5%) [54]. It should be noted that weight loss is not once and for all. After successful weight loss, it is necessary to adhere to a healthy lifestyle to prevent recurrence.

5.2 Psychological intervention and compliance improvement

Lifestyle intervention requires high compliance from patients, which is also a difficulty in implementation. There may be the following reasons for poor patient compliance: (1) lack of motivation and vague goals, which show that patients lack internal motivation (such as “no sense of urgency in asymptomatic period”) or the goal setting is too general (such as “eat less and move more”); (2) limited time and resources, which show that it is difficult for busy people to exercise regularly, and those with limited economic conditions cannot afford healthy food or gym fees; (3) lack of knowledge and cognitive bias, manifested as misunderstanding of dietary principles (such as "sugar-free food can be eaten at will") or underestimating the risk of disease ("fatty liver is not a serious illness"); (4) lack of social support, manifested as uncooperative family members (such as continuing to cook high-fat meals) and interference from bad habits in social circles (drinking and gathering); (5) psychological and emotional disorders, which show that patients with anxiety or depression give up their diet plan because of emotional eating, and perfectionists give up completely after occasionally violating the rules; (6) physical discomfort and frustration, manifested as muscle aches after initial exercise and gastrointestinal discomfort caused by dietary changes (such as abdominal distension caused by a high-fiber diet).

Compliance may be improved in the following ways:

1. Clarify the motivation and goal: First, wake up the intrinsic motivation by understanding the benefits of lifestyle intervention to the body; Then gradually start from the specific goal: transform "losing weight" into "walking fast for 30 minutes three times a week and adding one vegetable to dinner" [55].

2. Reasonable planning: A single long-term training can be replaced by fragmented exercise (such as short-term stretching exercise). Eggs are used instead of salmon, and family weight training is used instead of gym training [56].

3. Timely positive feedback and understanding: During this period, if we face up to clinical data such as liver ultrasound images, we can show the changes of fatty liver by contrast and strengthen the disease cognition. At the same time, it positively guides patients to treat them positively, such as dispelling patients' view that failure once equals failure [57].

4. Family support: Patients' families can participate in a low-fat diet together, organize family exercise days with patients, and improve patients' compliance [58].

5. Psychological intervention: Guide patients to pay attention to the hunger-satiety signal and reduce emotional eating, especially the depression caused by insufficient positive feedback in the process, which should be noticed and intervened in in time [59].

6. Gradual adjustment and adaptation: starting with increasing one cup of water and reducing one spoon of oil every day, gradually transition to comprehensive diet adjustment; Adopt low-intensity exercise at the beginning, gradually increase the resistance ratio, and persist for a long time [60].

With the development of information technology, smart wearable devices can be used for long-term feedback, using an app to record diet/exercise (such as MyFitnessPal), and setting up an automatic reminder and achievement reward mechanism. Wearable devices (smartwatches) monitor heart rate and steps in real time and provide immediate feedback. For example, research has found that wearable devices can help patients easily track body data and promote a healthier and more active life [61]. It should be noted that being sedentary is also the main inducement of MASLD [62]. In modern society, most people are sedentary in their work and life, and smart devices can detect their sitting time and remind them.

6. Consideration of cultural factors and individual differences

6.1 Effects of dietary habits and cultural background on intervention effects

Lifestyle interventions are the cornerstone of MASLD management. Besides, the dietary modification is the most effective strategy [58]. However, the success of dietary interventions in the population is not consistent. An often underappreciated but critical factor influencing therapeutic outcomes is the patient's dietary habits and cultural background.

Dietary habits are deeply influenced by cultural, regional, and religious traditions. On the one hand, the Mediterranean diet, which is rich in fruits, vegetables, legumes, whole grains, and olive oil, is considered highly beneficial for the prevention and management of MASLD [35]. The southern European people naturally adhere to such a pattern, which is congruent with the recommended dietary approach for MASLD patients [59]. On the other hand, traditional East Asian diets, characterized by high consumption of rice, vegetables, fermented foods, and fish, generally exhibit a lower fat content and high fiber intake, which may also exert protective effects against hepatic steatosis [60, 61]. However, the rapid pace of urbanization and globalization has led to a nutrition transition in many regions [62]. Western dietary patterns—characterized by high intake of processed foods, added sugars, saturated fats, and red meats—have increasingly infiltrated regions with previously healthier eating traditions [63]. This nutritional transition has been a major driver of the increasing incidence of MASLD in non-Western countries, often coexisting with persistent cultural food preferences that may either conflict with or support modern dietary interventions [64].

Cultural perceptions of food are significantly influenced by dietary recommendations. For instance, in some Middle Eastern and South Asian cultures, abundant food and a larger body size are historically associated with wealth and health, potentially reducing motivation to adopt calorie-restricted diets [65]. Conversely, certain cultures emphasize communal meals and shared dishes, which can make individual dietary control more challenging. Furthermore, religious practices such as fasting (e.g., Ramadan in Islam, Lent in Christianity, or fasting in Buddhism) influence not only meal timing but also food choices [66]. These practices may interact with metabolic processes and, depending on their implementation, either benefit or exacerbate MASLD. For example, time-restricted feeding during fasting periods has been shown in some studies to improve metabolic markers; however, excessive caloric intake during non-fasting hours may negate such benefits [67]. Understanding and respecting these cultural dynamics are essential when designing patient-centered dietary interventions. Culturally tailored counseling and meal planning that integrates traditional foods and preparation methods can enhance patient engagement and compliance [68]. Another critical element influencing dietary intervention outcomes is nutritional literacy, which varies significantly across cultural and socioeconomic contexts [69]. Individuals with limited understanding of nutrition may misinterpret or be unaware of the health implications of their diet. Additionally, some cultures may lack equivalent terms for medical concepts like "insulin resistance" or "fatty liver," complicating education and communication efforts [70].

Dietary habits and cultural background play a crucial role in the effectiveness of lifestyle interventions in MASLD. A nuanced understanding of these factors enables healthcare professionals to deliver more effective, sustainable, and culturally resonant care. As the global burden of MASLD grows, so too must our capacity to individualize treatment strategies in a way that respects and integrates the lived experiences of patients from all cultural backgrounds [71].

6.2 Differences in health beliefs and acceptance among different groups of people

Differences in cultural values, socioeconomic conditions, education level, and exposure to health information all contribute to how individuals assess the seriousness of MASLD, their perceived vulnerability to the disease, and the perceived benefits of lifestyle modification or pharmacological therapy.

Cultural perceptions also shape treatment acceptance. In some communities, where obesity is not culturally stigmatized or recognized as a health risk, the early stages of MASLD are underrecognized until complications arise [72]. Gender roles may further influence how individuals engage with healthcare systems—men in certain societies may be less likely to seek preventive care, while women may encounter social or familial constraints that limit their ability to adopt personalized dietary and activity plans [73]. These context-specific factors underscore the importance of culturally sensitive educational approaches in MASLD management. Treatment outcomes can be significantly improved when healthcare professionals align their communication with the patient's belief systems. Approaches such as motivational interviewing, community-driven health education, and the integration of culturally resonant practices have demonstrated efficacy in enhancing treatment uptake and long-term adherence [74]. Ultimately, aligning clinical recommendations with patients' values and perceptions is vital for achieving sustainable improvements in MASLD outcomes.

7. Multidisciplinary team cooperation and clinical integration

7.1 Collaborative model of nutrition, exercise, psychology, and medicine

MASLD is a lifestyle-related condition that demands a multidisciplinary approach for optimal management. Traditional models relying solely on pharmacological treatment or physician-led counseling often fail to produce sustainable outcomes [75]. Recent evidence suggests that collaborative care models—incorporating nutritionists, exercise specialists, psychological counselors, and clinicians—can significantly improve both adherence and long-term effectiveness of MASLD interventions [76].

Nutritionists play a foundational role by offering personalized dietary plans that align with the patient's metabolic profile, comorbidities, and cultural eating habits. Their guidance helps patients adopt sustainable changes in calorie intake, macronutrient balance, and meal timing—factors crucial for reducing hepatic fat accumulation [77]. Exercise specialists, on the other hand, tailor physical activity programs to individual fitness levels and preferences. Structured aerobic and resistance training not only facilitates weight loss but also improves insulin sensitivity and liver enzyme profiles [78]. Psychological counselors help manage frequently overlooked factors such as emotional eating, low motivation, and mental health disorders, including depression and anxiety, which frequently co-occur with MASLD. Cognitive-behavioral strategies, motivational interviewing, and stress management techniques can enhance patients' readiness for change and long-term adherence to lifestyle interventions. Clinicians serve as coordinators, integrating diagnostic insight, pharmacotherapy when needed, and continuous medical monitoring to guide the overall care plan [79]. The synergy among these professionals allows for a patient-centered, holistic approach that goes beyond isolated interventions. Regular interdisciplinary meetings, shared electronic health records, and aligned treatment objectives ensure continuity of care and reduce conflicting advice. Evidence indicates that such integrated models lead to greater reductions in hepatic steatosis, improved cardiometabolic markers, and higher patient satisfaction rates compared to standard care [80].

In conclusion, a collaborative care framework that actively involves nutrition, physical activity, mental health, and clinical medicine offers a promising path for enhancing MASLD treatment outcomes. Future healthcare systems should prioritize integrated delivery models to address the complex behavioral and metabolic dimensions of MASLD.

7.2 The outpatient intervention pathway is linked to community resources

Effective management of MASLD demands a shift from episodic clinical care; it necessitates a structured, continuous intervention model that extends beyond the clinic. Outpatient-based intervention pathways, when linked effectively with community health resources, have demonstrated improved adherence, metabolic outcomes, and patient engagement in MASLD care [81]. In the outpatient setting, early risk stratification and personalized treatment plans form the foundation of intervention. These typically encompass lifestyle counseling, regular biomarker assessment, and the initiation of pharmacologic therapies when indicated [82]. However, without continuity of support, especially in lifestyle modification, patient dropout rates remain elevated. To address this gap, integrating outpatient care with community-based resources—such as local dietitians, exercise programs, mental health services, and digital health platforms—has emerged as a promising strategy [83, 84]. Community resource linkage enhances the scalability and sustainability of MASLD interventions. For example, referral systems connecting patients to local fitness centers or subsidized nutrition workshops help ensure that patients can act on clinical advice in their daily environments. Furthermore, collaboration with community health workers or peer support groups offers culturally relevant education and motivation, particularly in underserved populations. These linkages not only reinforce behavior change but also foster a sense of accountability and shared progress [85].

Digital tools also serve as an extension of outpatient care, enabling remote monitoring, virtual coaching, and real-time feedback. When aligned with community services and clinical oversight, these platforms help bridge logistical barriers and maintain patient engagement between clinic visits. The integration of outpatient pathways with community resources leads to a more comprehensive, ecosystem-based approach to MASLD management. Studies have shown that such coordinated care models can improve liver enzyme profiles, reduce hepatic fat content, and enhance patient satisfaction. Importantly, they also help address social determinants of health that are often barriers to successful MASLD treatment [86].

In conclusion, linking structured outpatient interventions with accessible, community-level resources plays a critical role in improving MASLD outcomes [87]. Healthcare systems should prioritize this integration to deliver more equitable, sustainable, and effective long-term care.

8. Clinical application tools and practice guidelines

8.1 Goal setting and individualized plan development

MASLD requires a patient-centered approach that emphasizes realistic and individualized goal setting [88]. Given the chronic and behavior-dependent nature of MASLD, traditional generic advice—such as "eat healthier" or "exercise more"—is often insufficient. Instead, structured frameworks such as SMART goals (Specific, Measurable, Achievable, Relevant, and Time-bound) are essential for creating clear, actionable, and sustainable treatment plans [89].

The initial phase of goal setting should be based on a comprehensive assessment of the patient's metabolic profile, comorbidities, psychosocial context, readiness to change, and available resources. Clinicians, together with patients, can co-develop personalized objectives that are both medically relevant and practically feasible. For example, rather than broadly recommending weight loss, a SMART goal might be: "Lose 5% of current body weight over the next 3 months through walking 30 minutes five times a week and reducing daily caloric intake by 500 kcal [90]." Importantly, goals should be revisited and adjusted regularly to reflect patient progress and evolving clinical needs. Continuous monitoring of anthropometric data, liver enzymes, and patient-reported outcomes helps in refining interventions and maintaining motivation. This iterative process encourages accountability while avoiding the discouragement that can result from overly ambitious targets [91].

Personalized planning also involves prioritizing the patient's preferences and cultural norms. A flexible approach might integrate dietary changes aligned with regional food habits or recommend physical activities that are enjoyable and accessible. In patients with psychological or socioeconomic barriers, including a mental health professional or social worker in the care team can help address nonmedical factors that hinder adherence [92].

Ultimately, SMART goals not only enhance communication between patients and providers but also increase the likelihood of long-term behavioral change—an essential element in reversing hepatic steatosis and improving metabolic outcomes. When paired with regular feedback and multidisciplinary support, individualized goal setting transforms MASLD care from a reactive model into a proactive, empowering process.

8.2 Monitoring metrics and follow-up recommendations

MASLD requires structured and evidence-based monitoring to assess disease progression, treatment response, and associated metabolic risk. Given the heterogeneity of MASLD—from simple steatosis to advanced fibrosis—the selection of appropriate monitoring parameters and timely follow-up is critical in preventing complications such as cirrhosis or hepatocellular carcinoma.

Key monitoring indicators include body weight, serum alanine aminotransferase (ALT), and liver imaging findings. Weight is a primary, modifiable risk factor and surrogate marker for therapeutic response [93]. A sustained weight loss of ≥5–10% is associated with histological improvement in steatosis and inflammation, and possibly fibrosis regression. Regular measurement of body mass index (BMI) and waist circumference at each follow-up visit offers insight into visceral adiposity, a key driver of hepatic lipid accumulation [94].

ALT and other liver enzymes (e.g., AST, GGT) are routinely used to monitor hepatic inflammation, though they lack specificity and may not accurately reflect histological changes in all patients. Nonetheless, downward trends in ALT—particularly when correlated with lifestyle modification—can indicate treatment efficacy [95]. For patients with persistently elevated transaminases or signs of liver dysfunction, further diagnostic evaluation is warranted.

Noninvasive liver imaging, such as ultrasound, transient elastography (FibroScan), or magnetic resonance imaging-proton density fat fraction (MRI-PDFF), plays an important role in both diagnosis and monitoring. Ultrasound is cost-effective for initial screening, while transient elastography provides a quantitative assessment of hepatic stiffness and steatosis, helping to detect fibrosis progression [96]. MRI-PDFF, though less accessible, offers a highly sensitive method to quantify liver fat and track longitudinal changes.

Follow-up intervals should be individualized based on disease severity, comorbidities (e.g., type 2 diabetes, cardiovascular disease), and treatment modality. For patients with early-stage MASLD and no advanced fibrosis, 6–12-month intervals may suffice [97]. Those with increased fibrosis risk or high ALT levels may require more frequent monitoring (every 3–6 months), particularly during initiation of therapeutic interventions [98].

A multidisciplinary follow-up plan—including input from hepatologists, primary care, dietitians, and physical activity specialists—is essential for ensuring adherence, tracking progress, and adjusting therapy [99]. Continuous monitoring using validated parameters helps clinicians detect early signs of disease progression and reinforces patient engagement in long-term care.

8.3 Clinical assessment tools and risk stratification

Effective clinical management of MASLD hinges on accurate assessment and risk stratification. Given the disease's broad clinical spectrum—from benign steatosis to progressive nonalcoholic steatohepatitis (NASH) and advanced fibrosis—early identification of high-risk individuals is essential to guide monitoring intensity and therapeutic interventions [100].

Initial evaluation of MASLD should begin with a comprehensive clinical history, including assessment of metabolic comorbidities such as obesity, type 2 diabetes mellitus (T2DM), hypertension, and dyslipidemia. Routine laboratory testing includes liver function tests (ALT, AST), fasting glucose, HbA1c, and lipid profile [101]. While elevated ALT is commonly used as a surrogate marker, many patients with advanced fibrosis may present with normal transaminase levels, underscoring the need for more sensitive tools [102].

Noninvasive fibrosis scoring systems are central to MASLD risk stratification. The Fibrosis-4 (FIB-4) Index and the NAFLD Fibrosis Score (NFS) are among the most widely used tools in both primary and specialty care. These scores incorporate age, liver enzymes, platelet count, and metabolic markers to estimate the likelihood of advanced fibrosis. Patients with low-risk scores can typically be managed in primary care, while those with indeterminate or high-risk scores may require referral for further evaluation [103].

Transient elastography (FibroScan) offers additional value by directly measuring liver stiffness and steatosis through controlled attenuation parameter (CAP). It is a noninvasive, reproducible tool that helps differentiate fibrosis stages and guide clinical decisions [104]. In some settings, magnetic resonance elastography (MRE) provides superior accuracy, particularly in obese patients, but is less accessible due to cost and availability [105].

Emerging tools, including serum biomarkers (e.g., PRO-C3, ELF test) and genetic risk scores, are being explored for enhanced prediction of disease progression, particularly in individuals with intermediate risk based on traditional algorithms [106]. Risk stratification is not static; it must be revisited regularly as the patient's metabolic profile, lifestyle, or treatment response evolves. A tiered approach—starting with simple scoring systems and escalating to advanced imaging or biopsy when indicated—maximizes resource efficiency while ensuring high-risk patients receive timely intervention [107].

Ultimately, integrating clinical assessment tools with a personalized, risk-based management plan is key to preventing MASLD-related complications and optimizing long-term outcomes.

9. Conclusions

As the cornerstone of the management of fatty liver disease (MASLD) associated with metabolic dysfunction, lifestyle intervention shows significant clinical value by directly targeting hepatic fat deposition and metabolic disorders. Based on the existing evidence, this chapter shows that the intervention strategy centered on diet optimization (such as the Mediterranean diet) and a personalized exercise program (combining aerobic and resistance training) cannot only effectively reduce the liver fat content and improve insulin sensitivity but also delay or even reverse the disease progress through moderate weight loss (5–10%). However, insufficient patient compliance and cultural background differences are still the main obstacles to long-term intervention. Therefore, integrating multidisciplinary team resources, adopting a patient-centered dynamic goal-setting framework, and combining with digital monitoring tools can enhance the feasibility and sustainability of intervention. In the future, it is necessary to further explore precise intervention models, such as nutrition stratification based on metabolic phenotype or exercise prescription optimization, and at the same time pay attention to the deep influence of socioeconomic factors on lifestyle changes so as to promote the transformation of MASLD management from "one size fits all" to an individualized and full-cycle care model.

Acknowledgements

This work was supported by the National Natural Science Foundation of China (Grant number 82303572). We would like this statement to appear in the acknowledgments section.

Conflict of interest

The authors declare no conflict of interest.

Author details

Yaoxin Wu[1], Huiling Gao[2], Chang Liu[3*] and Shan Gao[3*]

1 Faculty of Medicine, Dalian University of Technology, Dalian, China

2 College of life and health sciences, Northeastern University, Shenyang, China

3 Department of Central Laboratory, Central Hospital of Dalian University of Technology, Dalian, China

*Address all correspondence to: liuch2024@dlut.edu.cn; laraine33@163.com

References

[1] Chan WK, Chuah KH, Rajaram RB, Lim LL, Ratnasingam J, Vethakkan SR. Metabolic dysfunction-associated steatotic liver disease (MASLD): A state-of-the-art review. Journal of Obesity & Metabolic Syndrome. 2023;**32**:197-213. DOI: 10.7570/jomes23052

[2] Targher G, Byrne CD, Tilg H. MASLD: A systemic metabolic disorder with cardiovascular and malignant complications. Gut. 2024;**73**:691-702. DOI: 10.1136/gutjnl-2023-330595

[3] Hutchison AL, Tavaglione F, Romeo S, Charlton M. Endocrine aspects of metabolic dysfunction-associated steatotic liver disease (MASLD): Beyond insulin resistance. Journal of Hepatology. 2023;**79**:1524-1541. DOI: 10.1016/j.jhep.2023.08.030

[4] Younossi ZM, Kalligeros M, Henry L. Epidemiology of metabolic dysfunction-associated steatotic liver disease. Clinical and Molecular Hepatology. 2025;**31**:S32-s50. DOI: 10.3350/cmh.2024.0431

[5] Machado MV. MASLD treatment-a shift in the paradigm is imminent. Frontiers in Medicine. 2023;**10**:1316284. DOI: 10.3389/fmed.2023.1316284

[6] Huttasch M, Roden M, Kahl S. Obesity and MASLD: Is weight loss the (only) key to treat metabolic liver disease? Metabolism: Clinical and Experimental. 2024;**157**:155937. DOI: 10.1016/j.metabol.2024.155937

[7] de Abreu J, Azulay RS, Rodrigues V, de Abreu SLL, da Glória TM, Pinheiro FCM, et al. Predictors of hepatic fibrosis in type 2 diabetes patients with metabolic-dysfunction-associated steatotic liver disease. Biomedicine. 2024;**12**(11):2542. DOI: 10.3390/biomedicines12112542

[8] Wu H, Wei J, Wang S, Chen L, Zhang J, Wang N, et al. Dietary pattern modifies the risk of MASLD through metabolomic signature. JHEP Reports: Innovation in Hepatology. 2024;**6**:101133. DOI: 10.1016/j.jhepr.2024.101133

[9] Dukewich M, Yuan L, Terrault NA. At the crossroads of health and disease: Consequences of fat in the liver. Annual Review of Physiology. 2025;**87**:325-352. DOI: 10.1146/annurev-physiol-022724-105515

[10] Singh S, Osna NA, Kharbanda KK. Treatment options for alcoholic and non-alcoholic fatty liver disease: A review. World Journal of Gastroenterology. 2017;**23**:6549-6570. DOI: 10.3748/wjg.v23.i36.6549

[11] Yan T, Yan N, Xia Y, Sawaswong V, Zhu X, Dias HB, et al. Hepatocyte-specific CCAAT/enhancer binding protein α restricts liver fibrosis progression. The Journal of Clinical Investigation. 2024;**134**(7):e166731. DOI: 10.1172/jci166731

[12] Bansal SK, Bansal MB. Pathogenesis of MASLD and MASH—Role of insulin resistance and lipotoxicity. Alimentary Pharmacology & Therapeutics. 2024;**59**(Suppl 1):S10-s22. DOI: 10.1111/apt.17930

[13] Moore MP, Cunningham RP, Meers GM, Johnson SA, Wheeler AA, Ganga RR, et al. Compromised hepatic mitochondrial fatty acid oxidation and reduced markers of mitochondrial turnover in human NAFLD. Hepatology (Baltimore, Md). 2022;**76**:1452-1465. DOI: 10.1002/hep.32324

[14] Zheng C, Wang L, Zou T, Lian S, Luo J, Lu Y, et al. Ileitis promotes MASLD

progression via bile acid modulation and enhanced TGR5 signaling in ileal CD8(+) T cells. Journal of Hepatology. 2024;**80**:764-777. DOI: 10.1016/j.jhep.2023.12.024

[15] Afonso MB, Islam T, Magusto J, Amorim R, Lenoir V, Simões RF, et al. RIPK3 dampens mitochondrial bioenergetics and lipid droplet dynamics in metabolic liver disease. Hepatology (Baltimore, Md). 2023;**77**:1319-1334. DOI: 10.1002/hep.32756

[16] Jiang X, Fulte S, Deng F, Chen S, Xie Y, Chao X, et al. Lack of VMP1 impairs hepatic lipoprotein secretion and promotes non-alcoholic steatohepatitis. Journal of Hepatology. 2022;**77**:619-631. DOI: 10.1016/j.jhep.2022.04.010

[17] Jiang X, Chen A, Ding WX, Ni HM. VMP1 regulates hepatic lipoprotein secretion and NASH independent of autophagy. Autophagy. 2023;**19**:367-369. DOI: 10.1080/15548627.2022.2080958

[18] Liu C, Zhou B, Meng M, Zhao W, Wang D, Yuan Y, et al. FOXA3 induction under endoplasmic reticulum stress contributes to non-alcoholic fatty liver disease. Journal of Hepatology. 2021;**75**:150-162. DOI: 10.1016/j.jhep.2021.01.042

[19] Deja S, Fletcher JA, Kim CW, Kucejova B, Fu X, Mizerska M, et al. Hepatic malonyl-CoA synthesis restrains gluconeogenesis by suppressing fat oxidation, pyruvate carboxylation, and amino acid availability. Cell Metabolism. 2024;**36**:1088-104.e12. DOI: 10.1016/j.cmet.2024.02.004

[20] Zhang Z, TeSlaa T, Xu X, Zeng X, Yang L, Xing G, et al. Serine catabolism generates liver NADPH and supports hepatic lipogenesis. Nature Metabolism. 2021;**3**:1608-1620. DOI: 10.1038/s42255-021-00487-4

[21] Phoolchund AGS, Khakoo SI. MASLD and the development of HCC: Pathogenesis and therapeutic challenges. Cancers. 2024;**16**(2):259. DOI: 10.3390/cancers16020259

[22] Wu Y, Tan Z, Zhen J, Liu C, Zhang J, Liao F, et al. Association between diet soft drink consumption and metabolic dysfunction-associated steatotic liver disease: Findings from the NHANES. BMC Public Health. 2023;**23**:2286. DOI: 10.1186/s12889-023-17223-0

[23] Mehmood R, Sheikh N, Khawar MB, Abbasi MH, Mukhtar M. High-fat diet intake ameliorates the expression of hedgehog signaling pathway in adult rat liver. Molecular Biology Reports. 2022;**49**:1985-1994. DOI: 10.1007/s11033-021-07012-6

[24] Demaria TM, Crepaldi LD, Costa-Bartuli E, Branco JR, Zancan P, Sola-Penna M. Once a week consumption of Western diet over twelve weeks promotes sustained insulin resistance and non-alcoholic fat liver disease in C57BL/6 J mice. Scientific Reports. 2023;**13**:3058. DOI: 10.1038/s41598-023-30254-2

[25] Brouwers B, Rao G, Tang Y, Rodríguez Á, Glass LC, Hartman ML. Incretin-based investigational therapies for the treatment of MASLD/MASH. Diabetes Research and Clinical Practice. 2024;**211**:111675. DOI: 10.1016/j.diabres.2024.111675

[26] Lian CY, Zhai ZZ, Li ZF, Wang L. High fat diet-triggered non-alcoholic fatty liver disease: A review of proposed mechanisms. Chemico-Biological Interactions. 2020;**330**:109199. DOI: 10.1016/j.cbi.2020.109199

[27] Sampaio LP. Ketogenic diet for epilepsy treatment. Arquivos de Neuro-Psiquiatria. 2016;**74**:842-848. DOI: 10.1590/0004-282x20160116

[28] El-Shafie AM, Bahbah WA, Abd El Naby SA, Omar ZA, Basma EM, Hegazy AAA, et al. Impact of two ketogenic diet types in refractory childhood epilepsy. Pediatric Research. 2023;**94**:1978-1989. DOI: 10.1038/s41390-023-02554-w

[29] Long F, Bhatti MR, Kellenberger A, Sun W, Modica S, Höring M, et al. A low-carbohydrate diet induces hepatic insulin resistance and metabolic associated fatty liver disease in mice. Molecular Metabolism. 2023;**69**:101675. DOI: 10.1016/j.molmet.2023.101675

[30] Barber TM, Kabisch S, Pfeiffer AFH, Weickert MO. The effects of the Mediterranean diet on health and gut microbiota. Nutrients. 2023;**15**(9):2150. DOI: 10.3390/nu15092150

[31] Miyazawa T, Burdeos GC, Itaya M, Nakagawa K, Miyazawa T. Vitamin E: Regulatory redox interactions. IUBMB Life. 2019;**71**:430-441. DOI: 10.1002/iub.2008

[32] Calder PC. Omega-3 fatty acids and inflammatory processes: From molecules to man. Biochemical Society Transactions. 2017;**45**:1105-1115. DOI: 10.1042/bst20160474

[33] Righetti M. Protective effect of vitamin B therapy on bone and cardiovascular disease. Recent Patents on Cardiovascular Drug Discovery. 2009;**4**:37-44. DOI: 10.2174/157489009787260061

[34] Liu J, Li C, Yang Y, Li J, Sun X, Zhang Y, et al. Special correlation between diet and MASLD: Positive or negative? Cell & Bioscience. 2025;**15**:44. DOI: 10.1186/s13578-025-01382-1

[35] Ueba Y, Ikeda K, Tabara Y, Nakayama T, Tanaka D, Takahashi Y, et al. Dietary patterns rich in soybean products, vegetables, fish, fruits, and miso soup were inversely associated with fatty liver index: The Nagahama study. Journal of Nutritional Science and Vitaminology. 2025;**71**:25-33. DOI: 10.3177/jnsv.71.25

[36] Jamil A, Chivese T, Elshaikh U, Sendall M. Efficacy of the Mediterranean diet in treating metabolic dysfunction-associated steatotic liver disease (MASLD) in children and adolescents: A systematic review and meta-analysis. BMC Public Health. 2024;**24**:2701. DOI: 10.1186/s12889-024-19378-w

[37] Clinton SK. Lycopene: Chemistry, biology, and implications for human health and disease. Nutrition Reviews. 1998;**56**:35-51. DOI: 10.1111/j.1753-4887.1998.tb01691.x

[38] Covas MI. Olive oil and the cardiovascular system. Pharmacological Research. 2007;**55**:175-186. DOI: 10.1016/j.phrs.2007.01.010

[39] Anderson JW, Johnstone BM, Cook-Newell ME. Meta-analysis of the effects of soy protein intake on serum lipids. The New England Journal of Medicine. 1995;**333**:276-282. DOI: 10.1056/nejm199508033330502

[40] White D. Healthy uses for garlic. The Nursing Clinics of North America. 2021;**56**:153-156. DOI: 10.1016/j.cnur.2020.12.001

[41] Mendivil CO. Dietary fish, fish nutrients, and immune function: A review. Frontiers in Nutrition. 2020;7:617652. DOI: 10.3389/fnut.2020.617652

[42] Gao Y, Zhang W, Zeng LQ, Bai H, Li J, Zhou J, et al. Exercise and dietary intervention ameliorate high-fat diet-induced NAFLD and liver aging by inducing lipophagy. Redox Biology.

2020;**36**:101635. DOI: 10.1016/j.redox.2020.101635

[43] Qian X, Wang T, Gong J, Wang L, Chen X, Lin H, et al. Exercise in mice ameliorates high-fat diet-induced nonalcoholic fatty liver disease by lowering HMGCS2. Aging. 2021;**13**:8960-8974. DOI: 10.18632/aging.202717

[44] Zou Y, Chen Z, Sun C, Yang D, Zhou Z, Peng X, et al. Exercise intervention mitigates pathological liver changes in NAFLD zebrafish by activating SIRT1/AMPK/NRF2 signaling. International Journal of Molecular Sciences. 2021;**22**(20):10940. DOI: 10.3390/ijms222010940

[45] Ezpeleta M, Gabel K, Cienfuegos S, Kalam F, Lin S, Pavlou V, et al. Effect of alternate day fasting combined with aerobic exercise on non-alcoholic fatty liver disease: A randomized controlled trial. Cell Metabolism. 2023;**35**:56-70.e3. DOI: 10.1016/j.cmet.2022.12.001

[46] Damasceno de Lima R, Fudoli Lins Vieira R, Rosetto Muñoz V, Chaix A, Azevedo Macedo AP, Calheiros Antunes G, et al. Time-restricted feeding combined with resistance exercise prevents obesity and improves lipid metabolism in the liver of mice fed a high-fat diet. American Journal of Physiology Endocrinology and Metabolism. 2023;**325**:E513-Ee28. DOI: 10.1152/ajpendo.00129.2023

[47] Gonzalez JT, Fuchs CJ, Betts JA, van Loon LJ. Liver glycogen metabolism during and after prolonged endurance-type exercise. American Journal of Physiology Endocrinology and Metabolism. 2016;**311**:E543-E553. DOI: 10.1152/ajpendo.00232.2016

[48] Yarizadeh H, Eftekhar R, Anjom-Shoae J, Speakman JR, Djafarian K. The effect of aerobic and resistance training and combined exercise modalities on subcutaneous abdominal fat: A systematic review and meta-analysis of randomized clinical trials. Advances in Nutrition (Bethesda, Md). 2021;**12**:179-196. DOI: 10.1093/advances/nmaa090

[49] Keating SE, Sabag A, Hallsworth K, Hickman IJ, Macdonald GA, Stine JG, et al. Exercise in the management of metabolic-associated fatty liver disease (MAFLD) in adults: A position statement from exercise and sport science Australia. Sports Medicine (Auckland, NZ). 2023;**53**:2347-2371. DOI: 10.1007/s40279-023-01918-w

[50] van der Velde J, Boone SC, Winters-van Eekelen E, Hesselink MKC, Schrauwen-Hinderling VB, Schrauwen P, et al. Timing of physical activity in relation to liver fat content and insulin resistance. Diabetologia. 2023;**66**:461-471. DOI: 10.1007/s00125-022-05813-3

[51] Gonzalez-Gil AM, Elizondo-Montemayor L. The role of exercise in the interplay between myokines, hepatokines, osteokines, adipokines, and modulation of inflammation for energy substrate redistribution and fat mass loss: A review. Nutrients. 2020;**12**(6):1899. DOI: 10.3390/nu12061899

[52] Wen X, Zhang B, Wu B, Xiao H, Li Z, Li R, et al. Signaling pathways in obesity: Mechanisms and therapeutic interventions. Signal Transduction and Targeted Therapy. 2022;7:298. DOI: 10.1038/s41392-022-01149-x

[53] Fogarasi A, Gonzalez K, Dalamaga M, Magkos F. The impact of the rate of weight loss on body composition and metabolism. Current Obesity Reports. 2022;**11**:33-44. DOI: 10.1007/s13679-022-00470-4

[54] Stine JG, DiJoseph K, Pattison Z, Harrington A, Chinchilli VM,

Schmitz KH, et al. Exercise training is associated with treatment response in liver fat content by magnetic resonance imaging independent of clinically significant body weight loss in patients with nonalcoholic fatty liver disease: A systematic review and meta-analysis. The American Journal of Gastroenterology. 2023;**118**:1204-1213. DOI: 10.14309/ajg.0000000000002098

[55] Naar S, Ellis D, Idalski Carcone A, Jacques-Tiura AJ, Cunningham P, Templin T, et al. Outcomes from a sequential multiple assignment randomized trial of weight loss strategies for African American adolescents with obesity. Annals of Behavioral Medicine: A Publication of the Society of Behavioral Medicine. 2019;**53**:928-938. DOI: 10.1093/abm/kaz003

[56] Iwanaga S, Hashida R, Takano Y, Bekki M, Nakano D, Omoto M, et al. Hybrid training system improves insulin resistance in patients with nonalcoholic fatty liver disease: A randomized controlled pilot study. The Tohoku Journal of Experimental Medicine. 2020;**252**:23-32. DOI: 10.1620/tjem.252.23

[57] Leng G, Adan RAH, Belot M, Brunstrom JM, de Graaf K, Dickson SL, et al. The determinants of food choice. The Proceedings of the Nutrition Society. 2017;**76**:316-327. DOI: 10.1017/s002966511600286x

[58] Mayberry LS, Osborn CY. Family support, medication adherence, and glycemic control among adults with type 2 diabetes. Diabetes Care. 2012;**35**:1239-1245. DOI: 10.2337/dc11-2103

[59] Yu J, Song P, Zhang Y, Wei Z. Effects of mindfulness-based intervention on the treatment of problematic eating behaviors: A systematic review. Journal of Alternative and Complementary Medicine (New York, NY). 2020;**26**:666-679. DOI: 10.1089/acm.2019.0163

[60] Yu-Poth S, Zhao G, Etherton T, Naglak M, Jonnalagadda S, Kris-Etherton PM. Effects of the national cholesterol education program's step I and step II dietary intervention programs on cardiovascular disease risk factors: A meta-analysis. The American Journal of Clinical Nutrition. 1999;**69**:632-646. DOI: 10.1093/ajcn/69.4.632

[61] Xu L, Zhou C, Ling Y, Ding H, Wang Q, Wu Y, et al. Effects of short-term unsupervised exercise, based on smart bracelet monitoring, on body composition in patients recovering from breast cancer. Integrative Cancer Therapies. 2021;**20**:15347354211040780. DOI: 10.1177/15347354211040780

[62] Kanuri G, Bergheim I. In vitro and in vivo models of non-alcoholic fatty liver disease (NAFLD). International Journal of Molecular Sciences. 2013;**14**:11963-11980. DOI: 10.3390/ijms140611963

[63] Armandi A, Bugianesi E. Dietary and pharmacological treatment in patients with metabolic-dysfunction associated steatotic liver disease. European Journal of Internal Medicine. 2024;**122**:20-27. DOI: 10.1016/j.ejim.2024.01.005

[64] Bernardino M, Sison NKD, Bruce JC, Tiribelli C, Rosso N. Understanding and exploring the food preferences of Filipino school-aged children through free drawing as a projective technique. Nutrients. 2024;**16**(23):4035. DOI: 10.3390/nu16234035

[65] Hallberg L, Björn-Rasmussen E, Garby L, Pleehachinda R, Suwanik R. Iron absorption from south-east Asian diets and the effect of iron fortification. The American Journal of Clinical Nutrition. 1978;**31**:1403-1408. DOI: 10.1093/ajcn/31.8.1403

[66] Zhang S, Huo Z, Borné Y, Meng G, Zhang Q, Liu L, et al. Adherence to a healthy lifestyle including sleep and sedentary behaviors and risk of metabolic dysfunction-associated steatotic liver disease in Chinese adults. Preventive Medicine. 2024;**184**:107971. DOI: 10.1016/j.ypmed.2024.107971

[67] Popkin BM, Adair LS, Ng SW. Global nutrition transition and the pandemic of obesity in developing countries. Nutrition Reviews. 2012;**70**:3-21. DOI: 10.1111/j.1753-4887.2011.00456.x

[68] Liu L, Nishihara R, Qian ZR, Tabung FK, Nevo D, Zhang X, et al. Association between inflammatory diet pattern and risk of colorectal carcinoma subtypes classified by immune responses to tumor. Gastroenterology. 2017;**153**:1517-30.e14. DOI: 10.1053/j.gastro.2017.08.045

[69] Lazarus JV, Mark HE, Allen AM, Arab JP, Carrieri P, Noureddin M, et al. A global action agenda for turning the tide on fatty liver disease. Hepatology. 2024;**79**:502-523. DOI: 10.1097/hep.0000000000000545

[70] Mora N, Golden SH. Understanding cultural influences on dietary habits in Asian, middle eastern, and Latino patients with type 2 diabetes: A review of current literature and future directions. Current Diabetes Reports. 2017;**17**:126. DOI: 10.1007/s11892-017-0952-6

[71] Miao L, Targher G, Byrne CD, Cao YY, Zheng MH. Current status and future trends of the global burden of MASLD. Trends in Endocrinology and Metabolism. 2024;**35**:697-707. DOI: 10.1016/j.tem.2024.02.007

[72] Almansour HA, Chaar B, Saini B. Pharmacists' perspectives about their role in care of patients with diabetes observing Ramadan. Research in Social & Administrative Pharmacy. 2017;**13**:109-122. DOI: 10.1016/j.sapharm.2016.02.006

[73] Jamshed H, Beyl RA, Della Manna DL, Yang ES, Ravussin E, Peterson CM. Early time-restricted feeding improves 24-hour glucose levels and affects markers of the circadian clock, aging, and autophagy in humans. Nutrients. 2019;**11**(6):1234. DOI: 10.3390/nu11061234

[74] Gkotzamanis V, Panagiotakos D. Dietary interventions and cognition: A systematic review of clinical trials. Psychiatriki. 2020;**31**:248-256. DOI: 10.22365/jpsych.2020.313.248

[75] Truman E, Lane D, Elliott C. Defining food literacy: A scoping review. Appetite. 2017;**116**:365-371. DOI: 10.1016/j.appet.2017.05.007

[76] Muñoz-Restrepo AM, Navas MC, Daza J, Girala M, Ridruejo E, Gerken G, et al. Prevention in hepatology. Journal of Personalized Medicine. 2024;**14**(2):132. DOI: 10.3390/jpm14020132

[77] Jespersen S, Fritt-Rasmussen A, Madsbad S, Pedersen BK, Krogh-Madsen R, Weis N. Prevalence of cardiometabolic co-morbidities in patients with vs persons without chronic hepatitis B: The FitLiver cohort study. World Journal of Hepatology. 2025;**17**:97797. DOI: 10.4254/wjh.v17.i1.97797

[78] Wohlgemuth KJ, Arieta LR, Brewer GJ, Hoselton AL, Gould LM, Smith-Ryan AE. Sex differences and considerations for female specific nutritional strategies: A narrative review. Journal of the International Society of Sports Nutrition. 2021;**18**:27. DOI: 10.1186/s12970-021-00422-8

[79] Morris LS, Grehl MM, Rutter SB, Mehta M, Westwater ML. On what motivates us: A detailed review of intrinsic v. extrinsic motivation. Psychological Medicine. 2022;**52**:1801-1816. DOI: 10.1017/s0033291722001611

[80] Lin W, Zheng W, Dai N, Wu Y, Zhang X. Neddylation and MASLD: From pathophysiology to therapy. Liver International. 2025;**45**:e70064. DOI: 10.1111/liv.70064

[81] El-Kassas M, Awad A, Elbadry M, Arab JP. Tailored model of care for patients with metabolic dysfunction-associated steatotic liver disease. Seminars in Liver Disease. 2024;**44**:54-68. DOI: 10.1055/a-2253-9181

[82] Reytor-González C, Annunziata G, Campuzano-Donoso M, Morales-López T, Basantes-Tituaña C, Fascì-Spurio F, et al. Endocrinologist's crucial role in metabolic dysfunction-associated steatotic liver disease: A comprehensive review. Minerva Endocrinol (Torino). 2025;**50**(2):209-226. DOI: 10.23736/s2724-6507.24.04314-8

[83] Zeng XF, Varady KA, Wang XD, Targher G, Byrne CD, Tayyem R, et al. The role of dietary modification in the prevention and management of metabolic dysfunction-associated fatty liver disease: An international multidisciplinary expert consensus. Metabolism. 2024;**161**:156028. DOI: 10.1016/j.metabol.2024.156028

[84] Taube M, Quentin W. Provision of community-based mental health care, Latvia. Bulletin of the World Health Organization. 2020;**98**:426-430. DOI: 10.2471/blt.19.239913

[85] Arold D, Bornstein SR, Perakakis N, Ehrlich S, Bernardoni F. Regional gray matter changes in steatotic liver disease provide a neurobiological link to depression: A cross-sectional UK biobank cohort study. Metabolism. 2024;**159**:155983. DOI: 10.1016/j.metabol.2024.155983

[86] Younossi ZM, Alqahtani SA, Alswat K, Yilmaz Y, Keklikkiran C, Funuyet-Salas J, et al. Global survey of stigma among physicians and patients with nonalcoholic fatty liver disease. Journal of Hepatology. 2024;**80**:419-430. DOI: 10.1016/j.jhep.2023.11.004

[87] Kendall TJ, Chng E, Ren Y, Tai D, Ho G, Fallowfield JA. Outcome prediction in metabolic dysfunction-associated steatotic liver disease using stain-free digital pathological assessment. Liver International. 2024;**44**:2511-2516. DOI: 10.1111/liv.16062

[88] Allen AM, Charlton M, Cusi K, Harrison SA, Kowdley KV, Noureddin M, et al. Guideline-based management of metabolic dysfunction-associated steatotic liver disease in the primary care setting. Postgraduate Medicine. 2024;**136**:229-245. DOI: 10.1080/00325481.2024.2325332

[89] Zhu G, Song Y, Lu Z, Yi Q, Xu R, Xie Y, et al. Machine learning models for predicting metabolic dysfunction-associated steatotic liver disease prevalence using basic demographic and clinical characteristics. Journal of Translational Medicine. 2025;**23**:381. DOI: 10.1186/s12967-025-06387-5

[90] Song SJ, Nogami A, Liang LY, Yoneda M, Leung HHW, Nakajima A, et al. Performance of continuous controlled attenuation parameter and liver stiffness measurement by the novel SmartExam in metabolic dysfunction-associated steatotic liver disease. Liver International. 2024;**44**:1167-1175. DOI: 10.1111/liv.15862

[91] Su TH, Yang SS, Lee MH, Kao WY, Huang SC, Chen FF, et al. High SAFE scores predict hepatocellular carcinoma in viral and non-viral hepatitis and metabolic dysfunction associated steatotic liver disease. Clinical and Molecular Hepatology. 2025:0118. DOI: 10.3350/cmh.2024.0822

[92] Anekwe CV, Jarrell AR, Townsend MJ, Gaudier GI, Hiserodt JM, Stanford FC. Socioeconomics of obesity. Current Obesity Reports. 2020;**9**:272-279. DOI: 10.1007/s13679-020-00398-7

[93] Dobbie LJ, Burgess J, Hamid A, Nevitt SJ, Hydes TJ, Alam U, et al. Effect of a low-calorie dietary intervention on liver health and body weight in adults with metabolic-dysfunction associated steatotic liver disease (MASLD) and overweight/obesity: A systematic review and meta-analysis. Nutrients. 2024;**16**(7):1030. DOI: 10.3390/nu16071030

[94] Hsu CC, Ness E, Kowdley KV. Nutritional approaches to achieve weight loss in nonalcoholic fatty liver disease. Advances in Nutrition. 2017;**8**:253-265. DOI: 10.3945/an.116.013730

[95] Wang X, Gao X, Wu R, Chi X, Xu H, Guan Y, et al. Serum qAnti-HBc combined with ALT and HBsAg predicts significant hepatic inflammation in HBeAg-positive immune active patients. Journal of Gastroenterology and Hepatology. 2022;**37**:1806-1814. DOI: 10.1111/jgh.15881

[96] Ozturk A, Olson MC, Samir AE, Venkatesh SK. Liver fibrosis assessment: MR and US elastography. Abdominal Radiology (NY). 2022;**47**:3037-3050. DOI: 10.1007/s00261-021-03269-4

[97] Tran SA, Le A, Zhao C, Hoang J, Yasukawa LA, Weber S, et al. Rate of hepatocellular carcinoma surveillance remains low for a large, real-life cohort of patients with hepatitis C cirrhosis. BMJ Open Gastroenterology. 2018;**5**:e000192. DOI: 10.1136/bmjgast-2017-000192

[98] Landsteiner A, Ullman K, Langsetmo L, Zerzan N, Kalinowski C, Haglund J, et al. VA Evidence-Based Synthesis Program Reports. Screening for Hepatocellular Carcinoma in Adults at Increased Risk. Washington (DC): Department of Veterans Affairs (US); 2023

[99] Zeng J, Fan JG, Francque SM. Therapeutic management of metabolic dysfunction associated steatotic liver disease. United European Gastroenterology Journal. 2024;**12**:177-186. DOI: 10.1002/ueg2.12525

[100] Tacke F et al. EASL-EASD-EASO clinical practice guidelines on the management of metabolic dysfunction-associated steatotic liver disease (MASLD). Journal of Hepatology. 2024;**81**:492-542. DOI: 10.1016/j.jhep.2024.04.031

[101] Newsome PN, Sanyal AJ, Engebretsen KA, Kliers I, Østergaard L, Vanni D, et al. Semaglutide 2.4 mg in participants with metabolic dysfunction-associated steatohepatitis: Baseline characteristics and design of the phase 3 ESSENCE trial. Alimentary Pharmacology & Therapeutics. 2024;**60**:1525-1533. DOI: 10.1111/apt.18331

[102] Smith A, Baumgartner K, Bositis C. Cirrhosis: Diagnosis and management. American Family Physician. 2019;**100**:759-770

[103] Abdelhameed F, Kite C, Lagojda L, Dallaway A, Chatha KK, Chaggar SS, et al. Non-invasive scores and serum biomarkers for fatty liver in the era of metabolic dysfunction-associated

steatotic liver disease (MASLD): A comprehensive review from NAFLD to MAFLD and MASLD. Current Obesity Reports. 2024;**13**:510-531. DOI: 10.1007/s13679-024-00574-z

[104] Loomba R, Ramji A, Hassanein T, Yoshida EM, Pang E, Schneider C, et al. Velacur ACE outperforms FibroScan CAP for diagnosis of MASLD. Hepatology Communications. 2024;**8**(4):e0402. DOI: 10.1097/hc9.0000000000000402

[105] Wei X, Qi S, Wei X, Qiu L, Du X, Liu Y, et al. Inflammation activity affects liver stiffness measurement by magnetic resonance elastography in MASLD. Digestive and Liver Disease. 2024;**56**:1715-1720. DOI: 10.1016/j.dld.2024.04.031

[106] Hegmar H, Wiggers T, Nasr P, Vessby J, Kechagias S, Nyhlin N, et al. Performance of novel collagen turnover biomarkers to detect increased liver stiffness in MASLD. Journal of Internal Medicine. 2024;**296**:177-186. DOI: 10.1111/joim.13813

[107] Zoncapè M, Liguori A, Tsochatzis EA. Non-invasive testing and risk-stratification in patients with MASLD. European Journal of Internal Medicine. 2024;**122**:11-19. DOI: 10.1016/j.ejim.2024.01.013

Chapter 5

Perspective Chapter: Targeting PTP1B for the Treatment of Steatosis – Insights from Viscosol's Role in Insulin-Mediated Lipid Metabolism Regulation

Muhammad Asim, Aleena Altaf, Aamir Sohail,
Maimoona Arshad, Faiza Noreen, Idrees Raza, Hamza Muneer,
Muhammad Murtaza Hasnain, Raza Sufyan and Imran Ullah

Abstract

Metabolic dysfunction-associated steatotic liver disease (MASLD), previously known as nonalcoholic fatty liver disease (NAFLD), involves excessive fat buildup in liver cells and is closely linked to insulin resistance, type 2 diabetes mellitus (T2DM), and dyslipidemia. This chapter discusses MASLD pathophysiology, focusing on disrupted lipid metabolism, inflammation, and the key role of protein tyrosine phosphatase 1B (PTP1B) in insulin signaling and metabolic balance. The high-fat diet (HFD) plus low-dose streptozotocin (STZ) mouse model mimics human T2DM and MASLD, showing hyperglycemia, lipid abnormalities, and liver fat accumulation. Viscosol, a flavonoid from *Dodonaea viscosa*, shows strong therapeutic potential as a PTP1B inhibitor. Given at 33 mg/kg intraperitoneally for 7 days, Viscosol improved insulin sensitivity by increasing insulin receptor (INSR), IRS1/2, PI3K, and AKT expression, and regulated lipid metabolism genes (SREBP1c, FAS, PPARγ). It lowered serum low density lipoprotein (LDL), very low-density lipoprotein (VLDL), and total cholesterol. Histology showed less liver fat, reduced fibrosis markers (α-SMA, TGF-β1), and decreased inflammation. Viscosol also boosted cholesterol efflux *via* ABCA1 and ApoA1 and lowered inflammatory cytokines (TNF-α, IL-6) and the oxidative stress marker FOXO1, restoring metabolic health. These results suggest Viscosol as a promising natural agent targeting PTP1B to treat insulin resistance, dyslipidemia, and hepatic steatosis in MASLD and T2DM. Further clinical studies are needed to confirm these effects in humans.

Keywords: PTP1B inhibition, MASLD, Viscosol, insulin resistance, dyslipidemia, hepatic steatosis

1. Introduction

Nonalcoholic fatty liver disease (NAFLD) is characterized by excessive fat accumulation (5–10%) in hepatic cells after excluding other liver disease causes like alcohol use and viral infections [1]. In hepatic steatosis, hepatocytes accumulate triacylglycerol (TAG)-rich lipid droplets, either microvesicular or macrovesicular, without accompanying inflammation or liver damage [2]. Simple steatosis is reversible with lifestyle changes such as diet and increased physical activity [2]. While initial TAG accumulation was thought to be hepatoprotective, excessive intrahepatic fat promotes disease progression [3]. Liver steatosis severity is classified into four grades based on fat percentage in liver cells: Grade 0 (<5%), Grade 1 (5–33%), Grade 2 (34–66%), and Grade 3 (>66%) [4].

1.1 Historical evolution of hepatic steatosis

Addison first described fatty liver in 1836 [5]. Later, similarities were found between liver changes in diabetic and obese patients and those with alcoholic liver disease [5]. In 1980, Ludwig et al. introduced the term nonalcoholic steatohepatitis (NASH) to describe a progressive fatty liver condition resembling alcoholic steatohepatitis [5]. The term "nonalcoholic fatty liver disease" (NAFLD) was coined by Schaffner and Thaler in 1986 [5].

1.2 Transition from NAFLD to MASLD

NAFLD has been redefined as metabolic dysfunction-associated liver disease (MASLD) to better reflect its metabolic basis. There is a bidirectional link between NAFLD and metabolic syndrome, each contributing to the other's development [5]. MASLD diagnosis requires hepatic steatosis plus one or more cardiometabolic risk factors: elevated BMI or waist circumference, impaired glucose metabolism, hypertension, high triglycerides, or low HDL-C [6].

1.3 Role of insulin resistance and dyslipidemia in MASLD

Key contributors to MASLD include obesity, type 2 diabetes mellitus (T2DM), hypertension, and dyslipidemia, all closely associated with insulin resistance [7, 8]. Peripheral insulin resistance in MASLD and MASH using hyperinsulinemic-euglycemic clamp has been demonstrated [8]. Insulin signaling impairments, especially involving insulin receptor substrate 2 (IRS2), are central to insulin resistance pathogenesis. MASLD rats exhibited increased fasting glucose and insulin, epididymal fat, hepatic steatosis, inflammation, and reduced IRS2 expression compared to controls [8]. Insulin resistance disrupts lipid metabolism, leading to MASLD. Visceral adiposity elevates pro-inflammatory cytokines such as TNF-α, IL-6, and IL-1β while reducing adiponectin, causing systemic insulin resistance [9]. Lipoprotein lipase (LPL) and hormone-sensitive lipase (HSL) regulate triglyceride and fatty acid metabolism; LPL hydrolyzes extracellular triglycerides, while HSL breaks down intracellular triglycerides in adipocytes. Insulin resistance increases HSL activity, releasing free fatty acids (FFA). Excess triglyceride storage in skeletal muscle is linked with insulin resistance due to reduced fatty acid oxidation and impaired FFA uptake, increasing serum FFAs [9].

High serum FFAs enter the liver, increasing very low-density lipoprotein (VLDL) production. Insulin resistance elevates FFA influx, reduces apolipoprotein B100 degradation, and increases apolipoprotein CIII expression. Microsomal triglyceride transfer protein (MTP) overexpression also raises VLDL production. SREBP-1c expression is increased, promoting fatty acid synthesis. Hepatic fatty acid metabolism is regulated by uptake, VLDL export, *de novo* synthesis (*via* SREBP-1c), and beta-oxidation. Fat accumulation in the liver is a hallmark of MASLD [8].

1.4 Epidemiology and global burden

MASLD prevalence is rapidly increasing, currently affecting approximately 40% of adults worldwide, projected to reach 55% by 2040. This rise corresponds with a two- to-three-fold increase in advanced liver diseases such as cirrhosis, hepatocellular carcinoma, and liver-related mortality. MASLD has surpassed alcoholic liver disease (ALD) as the leading cause of liver cirrhosis and is expected to become the primary cause of liver-related deaths globally [10]. MASLD and T2DM frequently coexist due to shared metabolic and biological pathways. Dyslipidemia, beta-cell dysfunction, and muscle loss significantly contribute to the development of both conditions. MASLD prevalence in T2DM patients ranges between 65% and 70%, reaching over 90% in studies utilizing liver biopsies for diagnosis [10]. NAFLD and NASH negatively affect patient-reported outcomes, including health-related quality of life and work productivity, worsening with disease progression. Patients report higher fatigue, depression, and anxiety compared to healthy populations [11].

1.5 Pathogenesis of hepatic lipid accumulation

1.5.1 Insulin resistance, oxidative stress, and inflammation

Insulin resistance (IR) is a common feature of NAFLD and metabolic syndrome. The two-hit hypothesis posits IR and fat accumulation as the first hit, followed by inflammation, hepatocyte injury, and fibrosis as the second hit, leading to NASH, cirrhosis, and hepatocellular carcinoma [12]. Obesity, a major cause of NAFLD, leads to fat deposition in adipose and hepatic tissue. Elevated FFAs cause lipotoxicity and adipose dysfunction. Dyslipidemia and IR stimulate pro-inflammatory cytokines like TNF-α, IL-1β, and IL-6, which inhibit insulin receptor signaling and reduce hepatic insulin sensitivity, promoting fibrosis and steatosis [12].

Redox reactions maintain hepatic physiological balance but are disturbed by excessive fat accumulation [13].

1.6 Role of *de novo* lipogenesis, mitochondrial dysfunction, and lipid droplet accumulation in hepatocytes

1.6.1 Transition from simple steatosis (NAFLD) to steatohepatitis (MASLD to MASH)

NASH is the progressive form of NAFLD, developing in about 20% of patients. Hepatic steatosis is the initial pathological event and represents the first hit in the double-hit theory, but alone it is insufficient to cause inflammation and fibrosis [14]. Disease progression involves additional factors, including oxidative stress, genetic variations, dyslipidemia, immune alterations, and gut microbiota changes. Dyslipidemia promotes fatty acid accumulation in the liver, causing steatosis. Oxidative stress, considered the second hit, arises from fatty acid oxidation, generating reactive oxygen species (ROS), lipid peroxidation, DNA damage, mitochondrial dysfunction, and increased pro-inflammatory cytokines. This results in hepatocellular injury, inflammation, and fibrosis [14]. The second hit theory is incomplete; a triple-hit model involving steatosis, lipotoxicity, and inflammation better explains NASH progression. Multiple inflammatory and immune pathways are activated during NASH, including TLR4 binding by free fatty acids, triggering NF-κB pathway and ER stress, and cytokine production such as TNF-α and IL-1β. T-cell activation, particularly Th17 and natural killer T cells, also increases in NASH livers [15].

1.7 Molecular mechanism of PTP1B in insulin signaling and insulin resistance

Insulin binding activates its receptor (INSR), leading to phosphorylation of downstream proteins IRS1 and IRS2. This activates the PI3K p85 subunit, which in turn activates AKT (PKB). Activated AKT facilitates GLUT4 vesicle translocation to the cell membrane *via* GTPase RAB10, enhancing insulin action and glucose uptake. Protein tyrosine phosphatase 1B (PTP1B), encoded by the PTPN1 gene (~50 kDa), is expressed in liver, adipose tissue, muscle, and brain. Its expression is upregulated by elevated free fatty acids, ER stress, and inflammatory signals. PTP1B inhibits insulin signaling by dephosphorylating IRS1 and INSR-beta, blocking the PI3K-AKT pathway [16].

1.8 Role of PTP1B in metabolic diseases

PTP1B overexpression reduces GLUT4 receptors on cell membranes, promoting hyperglycemia and contributing to type 2 diabetes. It drives insulin resistance, obesity, and T2DM, which are key factors in MASLD progression. Downregulating PTP1B reduces ER stress and halts MASLD advancement. Additionally, PTP1B overexpression causes leptin resistance, leading to obesity [17]. Human studies show elevated PTP1B protein and gene expression in skeletal muscle, liver, and adipose tissue of diabetic, obese, and insulin-resistant subjects. The PTP1B gene is located at chromosome 20q13, linked to insulin resistance, T2DM, and obesity. PTP1B knockout mice demonstrate resistance to weight gain, improved insulin sensitivity, reduced adipocyte mass, better glucose tolerance, and prevention of beta-cell destruction and diabetes onset [18].

1.9 Therapeutic potential of PTP1B inhibition

PTP1B's critical role in insulin signaling makes it a promising target for T2DM and MASLD therapy. However, challenges in targeting PTP1B include its positively charged active site, poor bioavailability, and selectivity issues. Consequently, few inhibitors reached clinical trials, and many were discontinued due to lack of efficacy [19]. *Dodonaea viscosa* (L.) is a flowering shrub genus with 60 species found in Australia, North America, South Africa, and South Asia. Traditionally, its extracts have been used to treat various diseases [20]. Viscosol contains flavonoids, terpenoids, saponins, phenolics, alkaloids, tannins, and C-alkylated flavonol derivatives. Its main anti-inflammatory compound is hautriwaic acid [20]. *D. viscosa* exhibits antidiabetic properties, confirmed by isolating nine components from Viscosol that inhibit PTP1B [21].

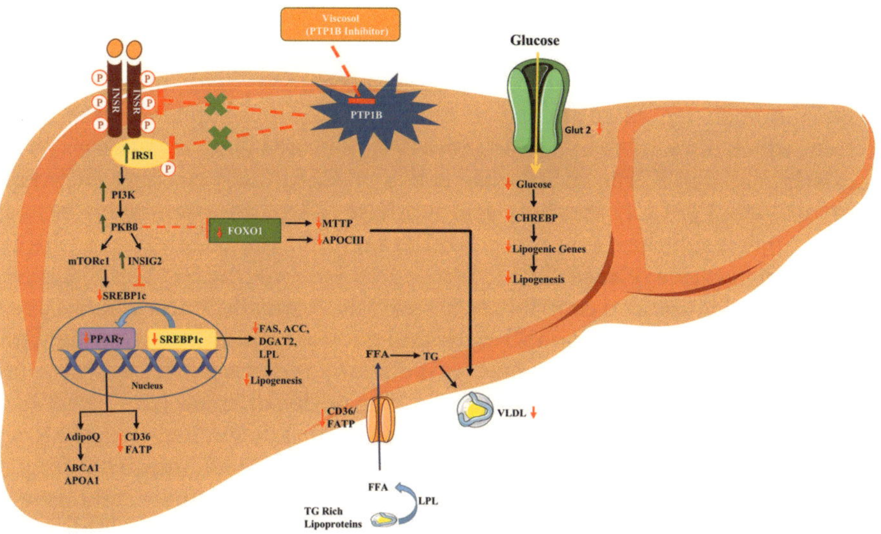

Figure 1.
Proposed molecular mechanism by which Viscosol inhibits PTP1B to improve insulin signaling, reduce lipogenesis, and restore lipid metabolism in MASLD.

As illustrated in **Figure 1**, Viscosol inhibits PTP1B activity, thereby enhancing insulin receptor signaling and downstream pathways that collectively reduce hepatic lipogenesis and improve lipid transport in MASLD (**Figure 1**). Studies report that *D. viscosa* has cytotoxic, anti-inflammatory, antioxidant, antibacterial, antiviral, hepatoprotective, and anti-hyperlipidemic activities [20].

1.10 Objective of this chapter

Since insulin resistance, obesity, and T2DM are root causes of MASLD, downregulating PTP1B expression can reverse these conditions. Viscosol inhibits PTP1B, thereby potentially reversing MASLD. It upregulates genes involved in glucose uptake and lipoprotein clearance, contributing to dyslipidemia reversal and improvement of hepatic steatosis.

2. Pathophysiology of hepatic steatosis and insulin resistance

2.1 Lipid accumulation and progression of hepatic steatosis

NAFLD is marked by lipid droplet (LD) accumulation in over 5% hepatocytes, known as steatosis. Insulin resistance (IR) drives lipid buildup and disease progression *via* multiple pathways. IR suppresses adipose tissue lipolysis, raising circulating nonesterified fatty acids (NEFAs), which the liver takes up and stores as triglycerides. Hyperinsulinemia stimulates hepatic *de novo* lipogenesis (DNL) through SREBP-1c activation. IR also reduces mitochondrial fatty acid oxidation and VLDL secretion, worsening intracellular fat accumulation [22]. Reactive lipids, such as diacylglycerols (DAG) and ceramides, accumulate, activating PKCε and impairing insulin receptor kinase activity, further disrupting insulin signaling. Lipotoxicity from these intermediates induces oxidative stress and inflammation, advancing steatosis [23].

2.1.1 De novo lipogenesis (DNL) and lipid droplet formation

Hepatic steatosis results from both adipose-derived fatty acids and DNL. DNL is transcriptionally regulated and driven by increased glucose uptake and insulin secretion, which upregulate lipogenic genes [24]. Elevated glucose enhances DNL *via* insulin-stimulated SREBP1c and glucose-activated ChREBP. Both enzymes, acetyl-CoA carboxylase 1 (ACC1) and fatty acid synthase (FAS), are essential for fatty acid synthesis. High insulin also suppresses FoxO1, a repressor of SREBP1c and ChREBP, promoting triglyceride storage [25].

Fatty acid oxidation also contributes to steatosis. Normally, mitochondria and peroxisomes perform β-oxidation. Genetic and environmental factors, along with IR, disrupt this process, leading to fat accumulation, microvesicular steatosis, and increased reactive oxygen species (ROS) that damage hepatocytes [26]. PPAR-α, abundant in the liver, regulates genes for fatty acid breakdown. Reduced PPAR-α activity suppresses enzymes, such as ACS, ACADs, and ACAA2, impairing fatty acid oxidation and promoting lipid buildup. This also disrupts carnitine metabolism, vital for mitochondrial fatty acid transport, and worsens oxidative stress by limiting ROS removal [27]. Low PPAR-α correlates with increased fat synthesis and reduced VLDL export, exacerbating NAFLD [28].

2.1.2 Transition from simple steatosis to steatohepatitis

Simple steatosis (NAFLD) initially protects hepatocytes by triglyceride storage. However, persistent fat leads to harmful lipid byproducts (DAG, ceramides), causing signaling disruption and oxidative stress. This triggers the release of danger-associated molecular patterns (DAMPs), initiating sterile inflammation [29]. Immune cells, such as Kupffer cells, macrophages, and neutrophils, infiltrate the liver, releasing cytokines (TNF-α, IL-6, MCP-1) that sustain chronic inflammation.

Chronic inflammation activates hepatic stellate cells (HSCs), which differentiate into myofibroblasts, producing excess extracellular matrix proteins. Fibrogenic signals such as TGF-β and Hedgehog molecules from damaged hepatocytes and liver sinusoidal endothelial cells (LSECs) drive fibrosis progression [30].

Fibrosis worsens as impaired autophagy in LSECs causes endothelial dysfunction, elevating NF-κB inflammatory signaling. This cycle of inflammation and hepatocyte death disrupts liver structure and function. Advanced glycation end products (AGEs) from chronic hyperglycemia bind to their receptor (RAGE) on the liver and immune cells, increasing oxidative stress and fibrosis. These processes collectively drive the shift from simple steatosis to steatohepatitis (NASH) [31].

2.2 Impaired lipoprotein metabolism and dyslipidemia

The liver regulates lipid homeostasis by synthesizing and secreting very low-density lipoproteins (VLDL) that transport triglycerides to tissues. In hepatic steatosis, this balance is disturbed by increased fatty acid delivery from adipose tissue, enhanced *de novo* lipogenesis (DNL), and reduced lipid processing or export *via* β-oxidation and VLDL secretion [32]. As a result, hepatic triglyceride synthesis surpasses VLDL export capacity, causing dyslipidemia characterized by high triglycerides, low HDL cholesterol, and increased small, dense LDL particles [33]. Though VLDL particle number may remain unchanged, their triglyceride content rises, promoting systemic hypertriglyceridemia and cholesterol-rich LDL formation through intravascular remodeling. Steatosis also impairs HDL metabolism, lowering HDL levels and altering particle size and composition [34].

2.2.1 Disrupted lipoprotein clearance

In hepatic steatosis, triglyceride-rich lipoproteins (TRLs) and remnants clear poorly due to altered receptor-mediated uptake and impaired lipid exchange [34]. Fatty liver cells express fewer LDL receptors (LDLR) because of increased PCSK9, elevating circulating atherogenic LDL [35]. High triglycerides activate cholesterol ester transfer protein (CETP), enriching LDL and HDL with triglycerides. Hepatic lipase then converts these small, dense LDL particles, which more easily penetrate arteries, and small HDL particles that are rapidly cleared by the kidneys, worsening dyslipidemia. Fibrosis in advanced steatosis further disrupts clearance by reducing hepatocyte function to produce VLDL and internalize lipoproteins [34].

2.2.2 Apolipoprotein B100 and microsomal triglyceride transfer protein (MTP)

Apolipoprotein B100 (ApoB100) is the main structural protein of LDL, VLDL, and IDL, essential for lipid transport from the liver to peripheral tissues [36]. MTP transfers triglycerides and phospholipids to ApoB100 during lipoprotein assembly, critical for VLDL formation. Disruption in ApoB100 or MTP leads to hepatic steatosis. MTP overexpression reduces hepatic triglycerides and steatosis [37]. Riboflavin deficiency impairs ApoB100 synthesis, lowering plasma lipoproteins and increasing hepatic lipid storage [38].

2.3 Inflammation, oxidative stress, and insulin resistance

2.3.1 Cytokine-mediated insulin resistance

Pro-inflammatory cytokines, such as TNF-α, IL-6, and MCP-1, released during cell stress, promote insulin resistance. TNF-α induces serine phosphorylation of IRS1, inhibiting its normal tyrosine phosphorylation, and activates JNK and IKKβ pathways, increasing oxidative stress and IR [39]. IL-6 upregulates SOCS-3, which blocks insulin receptor and IRS1 phosphorylation. TNF-α also stimulates IL-6, amplifying inflammation [40]. MCP-1 recruits macrophages to adipose tissue, reducing insulin-stimulated glucose uptake and suppressing adipogenic genes GLUT-4 and PPAR-γ, leading to lipotoxicity. It also disrupts hepatic insulin suppression of glucose production, raising hepatic triglycerides and steatosis [41].

2.3.2 JNK-NF-κB activation and lipotoxicity

Inflammation activates JNK in insulin-sensitive tissues, phosphorylating IRS1/2 at serine/threonine sites, disrupting PI3K-AKT signaling. This reduces GLUT4 translocation and suppresses gluconeogenesis, causing hyperglycemia and hyperinsulinemia. JNK also triggers NF-κB and AP-1, increasing inflammation and oxidative stress [42]. Mitochondrial dysfunction due to oxidative stress impairs fatty acid breakdown, causing lipotoxicity and increased ROS. ROS-JNK crosstalk promotes lipid peroxidation and ER stress, inducing apoptotic genes and cell death [43]. Persistent JNK and

NF-κB activation leads to hepatocyte death. DAMPs from dying cells activate hepatic stellate cells (HSCs), increasing collagen and extracellular matrix deposition, promoting fibrosis and, eventually, cirrhosis [44].

2.4 PTP1B: A key regulator in hepatic insulin resistance

Protein tyrosine phosphatase 1B (PTP1B), encoded by PTPN1, is a 50 kDa non-receptor phosphatase regulating multiple signaling pathways including insulin, leptin, and EGF [45]. Tissue-specific effects of PTP1B inhibition are shown in models. Skeletal muscle PTP1B deletion enhances insulin sensitivity by increasing phosphorylation of IR, IRS1, AKT, ERK1/2, and PI3K activity, without affecting lipid profile or adiposity [46]. Adipose-specific deletion increases adipocyte size, leptin, and lipogenesis while maintaining body weight [47]. In the liver, PTP1B deletion improves insulin sensitivity, suppresses gluconeogenesis and lipogenesis, and reduces ER stress by lowering p38-MAPK, JNK phosphorylation, and ER-stress markers PERK and eIF2α, improving lipid profile without changing body weight or adiposity [48]. **Figure 2** illustrates how overexpression of PTP1B disrupts insulin receptor signaling and glucose uptake, whereas inhibition of PTP1B by Viscosol restores the PI3K-AKT pathway and facilitates GLUT4 translocation, improving insulin sensitivity (**Figure 2**).

2.4.1 PTP1B's effect on insulin receptor and IRS pathway

Normally, insulin binds IR, triggering autophosphorylation and phosphorylation of IRS1/2, activating PI3K. PI3K's regulatory (p85) and catalytic (p110) subunits phosphorylate phosphoinositides, converting PIP2 to PIP3. This activates AKT, promoting protein synthesis, survival, and GLUT4 translocation for glucose uptake. PTP1B negatively regulates by dephosphorylating IR, IRS1, and IRS2, dampening PI3K/AKT signaling [49]. **Table 1** summarizes the contrasting roles of PTP1B activation and inhibition on insulin

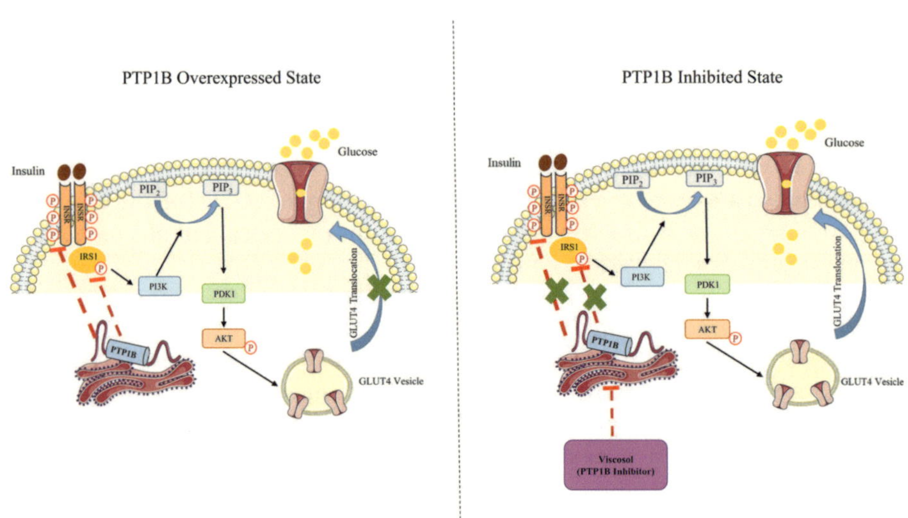

Figure 2.
Schematic representation of PTP1B's role in insulin signaling depicting impaired signaling in PTP1B overexpression versus restoration of insulin pathway upon PTP1B inhibition by Viscosol.

Aspect	PTP1B activation	PTP1B inhibition
Insulin signaling	Dephosphorylates insulin receptor (IR) and IRS, leading to insulin resistance.	Enhances insulin sensitivity by maintaining phosphorylation of IR and IRS.
Glucose homeostasis	Impairs insulin-mediated suppression of gluconeogenesis, contributing to hyperglycemia.	Improves glucose uptake, reduces hepatic gluconeogenesis, and lowers blood glucose levels.
Leptin signaling	Dephosphorylates JAK2, leading to leptin resistance and increased food intake.	Enhances leptin sensitivity, reducing food intake, and increasing energy expenditure.
Lipid metabolism	Promotes hepatic lipid accumulation and lipogenesis, contributing to MASLD.	Reduces hepatic fat accumulation by promoting fatty acid oxidation and inhibiting lipogenesis.
Potential therapeutic impact	Worsens metabolic disorders like type 2 diabetes and MASLD.	Shows promise as a target for drug development in insulin resistance, MASLD, and obesity.

Table 1.
Comparison of the metabolic effects and signaling pathways regulated by PTP1B activation versus inhibition.

signaling, glucose homeostasis, leptin sensitivity, lipid metabolism, and their implications for metabolic diseases such as MASLD and type 2 diabetes.

3. Experimental model and methodology

3.1 High-fat diet (HFD)-streptozotocin (STZ) induced diabetic mice model

3.1.1 Model justification

The high-fat diet (HFD) combined with low-dose STZ is a well-established mouse model that closely mimics human T2DM and MASLD. It replicates key features such as persistent hyperglycemia, insulin resistance, dyslipidemia, and hepatic steatosis. Unlike genetic models, this model includes environmental factors such as diet-induced obesity and β-cell damage, allowing better study of metabolic dysfunction and therapeutic testing [50].

3.1.2 Control vs. diabetic groups

Two groups were used: control mice on a standard diet with saline, and diabetic mice fed HFD plus low-dose STZ (40 mg/kg i.p. for 5 days) to impair β-cells. Diabetic mice showed hyperglycemia (>250 mg/dL fasting glucose), raised serum triglycerides, cholesterol, VLDL, LDL, and altered HDL. Histology revealed enlarged adipocytes with bigger lipid droplets, macrophage infiltration, and hepatic steatosis with lipid buildup and hepatocyte dilation [50]. This confirms the model's validity for T2DM and lipid metabolism studies.

3.2 Viscosol compound: Extraction and administration

3.2.1 Chemical properties and bioavailability

Viscosol (5,7-dihydroxy-3,6-dimethoxy-2-(4-methoxy-3-(3-methylbut-2-enyl) phenyl)-4H-chromen-4-one) is a flavonoid from *Dodonaea viscosa*, traditionally used for hyperglycemia and lipid disorders [50]. It potently inhibits PTP1B, a negative insulin signaling regulator involved in T2DM. Extraction follows standard phytochemical protocols, ensuring purity. Like many flavonoids, Viscosol has poor water solubility and faces metabolic degradation, requiring careful formulation for effective dosing.

3.2.2 Dosage and treatment

Viscosol was given at 33 mg/kg (~1 mg/mouse) *via* intraperitoneal injection dissolved in 1% DMSO. The treatment started after diabetes induction and lasted 7 days, monitoring fasting glucose and lipid profiles. This does align with prior studies showing insulin signaling and lipid metabolism improvements without toxicity [50].

3.3 Key biomarker analysis

3.3.1 Serum lipid profiling

Serum lipids were measured by enzymatic assays: triglycerides, total cholesterol (TC), LDL, VLDL, and HDL. Diabetic mice had high triglycerides, TC, LDL-C, and VLDL-C, with paradoxically raised HDL-C, typical of T2DM dyslipidemia. Viscosol treatment significantly lowered atherogenic lipoproteins and normalized HDL, showing its hypolipidemic effect [50].

3.3.2 Gene expression (RT-qPCR)

RT-qPCR quantified key insulin signaling and lipid metabolism genes in adipose and liver tissues. Targets included INSR, IRS1, IRS2, PI3K, SREBP1c, FAS, and PPARγ. Viscosol increased INSR, IRS1/2, and PI3K expression, indicating better insulin sensitivity. Lipogenic genes SREBP1c and FAS were up in adipocytes but down in hepatocytes, showing tissue-specific effects that reduce liver fat. PPARγ was upregulated in adipose, promoting healthy fat cell differentiation [50].

3.3.3 Histology (H&E and Oil Red O)

H&E and Oil Red O staining assessed adipose and liver morphology and lipid accumulation. Controls showed normal cell structure with minimal lipid. Diabetic mice had enlarged adipocytes, increased lipid droplets, macrophage infiltration, and clear hepatic steatosis with disrupted hepatocytes. Viscosol treatment restored normal cell morphology, reduced fat accumulation, confirming its hepatoprotective and anti-steatotic roles [50].

3.4 High-fat diet (HFD)-streptozotocin (STZ) diabetic mice model

3.4.1 Model justification

The HFD combined with the low-dose STZ mouse model replicates T2DM and MASLD well. HFD induces obesity and insulin resistance by fat buildup in the liver and adipose tissue, while STZ selectively damages pancreatic β-cells, reducing insulin secretion. This dual mechanism mimics human T2DM and MASLD effectively, making it ideal for testing treatments [50].

3.4.2 Control vs. diabetic groups

Control mice had a normal diet and saline injections. Diabetic mice on HFD plus STZ showed increased body weight, high fasting glucose, dyslipidemia (high triglycerides, cholesterol, LDL), and hepatic steatosis with enlarged adipocytes and inflammation. These changes mirror human diabetic and liver disease features [50].

3.5 Viscosol compound: Extraction and administration

3.5.1 Chemical properties and bioavailability

Viscosol, a flavonoid from *Dodonaea viscosa*, has strong anti-inflammatory, antidiabetic, and liver-protective effects. It inhibits PTP1B, which negatively affects insulin signaling. Like many flavonoids, it has low solubility and is prone to metabolic breakdown, requiring careful formulation for effective dosing [50].

3.5.2 Dosage and treatment

Viscosol was given intraperitoneally at 33 mg/kg (~1 mg/mouse) for 7 days after diabetes induction. Blood glucose and lipid levels were monitored to evaluate their effect on insulin sensitivity and lipid metabolism [50].

3.6 Key biomarker analysis

Serum lipids were measured enzymatically. Diabetic mice had high triglycerides, total cholesterol, LDL, and VLDL, with altered HDL. Viscosol treatment lowered these atherogenic lipids and normalized HDL, showing improved lipid metabolism [50].

3.6.1 Gene expression (RT-qPCR)

RT-qPCR assessed insulin signaling and lipid metabolism genes in adipose and liver tissues. Viscosol increased INSR, IRS1/2, PI3K, and AKT expression, improving insulin sensitivity. Lipogenic genes (SREBP1c, FAS, ACC) decreased in the liver but increased in adipose tissue, suggesting better lipid balance. PPARγ was upregulated in adipose, supporting healthy fat cell function [50]. Histology showed normal adipocytes and liver controls. Diabetic mice had enlarged fat cells, lipid droplets, macrophage infiltration, and liver steatosis with disrupted hepatocytes. Viscosol treatment reduced fat buildup and inflammation, restoring normal tissue structure, confirming its protective role [50].

4. Results and findings

4.1 Improvement in lipid profile and reduction in hepatic steatosis

4.1.1 Lipid biomarker changes

Treatment with Viscosol significantly improved serum lipid profiles in HFD-STZ diabetic mice. Levels of LDL, VLDL, and total cholesterol were notably reduced compared to untreated diabetic controls [50]. This lipid-lowering effect supports better insulin signaling and lipid metabolism, as shown by gene expression and histology data [50, 51]. These changes help reduce cardiovascular risks commonly seen in diabetes.

4.1.2 Cholesterol efflux enhancement

Viscosol also enhanced cholesterol efflux by increasing the expression of ABCA1 and ApoA1, key proteins involved in transporting cholesterol to HDL particles [51]. This improves reverse cholesterol transport, protecting cells from lipid toxicity and reducing atherosclerosis risk.

4.2 Histological changes in liver and adipose tissue

Histological analysis (H&E and Oil Red O staining) showed that Viscosol lowered lipid droplet accumulation in liver tissues. Diabetic mice had severe steatosis and disrupted liver cell structure, but treatment reduced fat buildup and improved liver morphology [50]. This aligns with its effect on genes regulating lipid metabolism.

Viscosol treatment also decreased fibrosis and inflammation markers like α-SMA and TGF-β1, leading to improved liver function tests (ALT, AST) [50, 51]. This confirms its protective effect against liver damage related to steatohepatitis and diabetes.

4.3 PTP1B inhibition restores insulin sensitivity

At the molecular level, Viscosol inhibited PTP1B, a negative regulator of insulin signaling. Expression of insulin receptor (INSR), IRS1, IRS2, PI3K, and AKT increased, improving glucose uptake and lowering blood glucose [50, 51]. This highlights the therapeutic potential of targeting PTP1B in insulin resistance. Chronic inflammation and oxidative stress contribute to insulin resistance. Viscosol significantly reduced pro-inflammatory cytokines TNF-α, IL-6, and oxidative stress marker FOXO1 in liver and adipose tissue [51]. This reduces inflammation, improves insulin sensitivity, and prevents tissue damage and fibrosis.

5. Synergy between Viscosol and GLP-1

The synergy between Viscosol (endoscopic gastric remodeling, EGR) and GLP-1 receptor agonists (GLP-1RA) comes from their combined effects on weight loss and liver health in MASLD patients with advanced fibrosis. EGR reduces stomach size, limits food intake, and slows digestion, while GLP-1RAs lower appetite, improve insulin sensitivity, and delay gastric emptying [52]. Together, they provide better weight reduction, improved liver fibrosis markers, and reduced insulin resistance than either alone. This combination offers an effective, less invasive treatment for complex metabolic liver disease cases.

5.1 Role of metformin in treating MASLD

Metformin improves insulin sensitivity, reduces liver glucose production, and modulates lipid metabolism. It activates AMPK, which lowers liver fat by blocking lipogenesis and increasing fatty acid oxidation. Metformin also reduces liver enzymes (ALT, AST), signaling less inflammation, and increases gut hormones like GLP-1 and

GDF15 that control appetite and metabolism [52]. It benefits gut microbiota, promoting metabolic health. Though histological improvements such as fibrosis reversal remain inconsistent, metformin is a cost-effective MASLD treatment, especially combined with drugs like GLP-1RAs.

5.2 SGLT2 inhibitor role in MASLD treatment

Originally for T2DM, SGLT2 inhibitors show promise in MASLD by enhancing insulin sensitivity and lowering blood glucose, thus preventing liver fat buildup. They also reduce liver inflammation and may slow fibrosis progression that leads to cirrhosis [52]. Their cardiovascular benefits are critical since MASLD increases heart disease risk. Although not yet officially approved for MASLD, early data suggest SGLT2 inhibitors could be valuable alongside standard liver therapies. **Table 2** highlights the clinical, pathological, and therapeutic differences between MASLD and MASH, emphasizing their progression from simple steatosis to inflammatory and fibrotic liver disease.

6. Advanced drug delivery systems using nanotechnology

6.1 Lipid-based nanoparticles

Micelles, liposomes, and lipid nanoparticles (LNPs) are favored for drug delivery due to biocompatibility and flexibility. Micelles effectively deliver hydrophobic drugs, liposomes carry both hydrophilic and hydrophobic agents, and LNPs protect nucleic acids with controlled release, critical for mRNA vaccines [53–55].

6.2 Polymeric drug delivery systems

Made from biodegradable polymers (PLGA, PLA, PEG), these nanoparticles allow controlled drug release. They can respond to stimuli like pH or reactive oxygen

Feature	MASLD (NASLD)	MASH (NASH)
Definition	Excess liver fat (≥5% of hepatocytes) without significant alcohol consumption.	Liver fat accumulated with inflammation and hepatocyte injury (ballooning), with or without fibrosis.
Pathogenesis	Insulin resistance, dyslipidemia, and metabolic dysfunction drive hepatic steatosis.	Chronic inflammation leads to hepatocyte damage, fibrosis, and potential progression to cirrhosis.
Histological features	Macro vesicular steatosis without significant inflammation or fibrosis.	Steatosis with hepatocyte ballooning, lobular inflammation, and fibrosis.
Metabolic associations	Strongly linked to obesity, type 2 diabetes (T2DM), and metabolic syndrome.	More severe metabolic dysfunction with increased risk of cardiovascular and liver-related mortality.
Treatment	Lifestyle modifications (diet, exercise), weight loss, metabolic control (e.g., GLP-1 RAs, SGLT2 inhibitors).	Same as MASLD, but with added focus on anti-inflammatory and antifibrotic strategies (e.g., obeticholic acid, FXR agonists).

Table 2.
Key distinctions between metabolic dysfunction-associated steatosis liver disease (MASLD) and metabolic dysfunction-associated steatohepatitis (MASH).

species (ROS) for targeted delivery. Examples include pH-sensitive polymers for tumors and dextran-based nanoparticles activated by ROS to enhance immune response [56, 57].

6.3 Peptide-based drug delivery systems

Short amino acid sequences target specific receptors, improving drug localization. EGFR-targeting peptides in liposomes treat lung cancer, and somatostatin-derived peptides target breast and prostate cancers. Recent peptides like RIPL increase selective uptake in cancer cells [17, 58, 59].

6.4 Inorganic nanoparticle-based systems

Dendrimers, mesoporous silica, magnetic, and gold nanoparticles offer high drug loading and targeting. Dendrimers encapsulate DNA and chemo drugs; magnetic nanoparticles are directed by external fields; gold nanoparticles are used in cancer photothermal therapy [18, 60, 61].

7. Targeted nanocarrier strategies to enhance Viscosol efficacy in MASLD

Modern delivery systems can boost Viscosol's bioavailability, liver targeting, and controlled release, enhancing its MASLD therapy potential. Lipid nanoparticles improve solubility and hepatic distribution, reducing side effects [62]. PEG-PLGA polymeric nanoparticles offer sustained release and protect Viscosol from degradation [56]. pH- or ROS-responsive carriers selectively release Viscosol in inflamed liver regions, increasing local drug levels while lowering toxicity [57]. Exosome-based delivery uses natural vesicles for precise liver targeting [63]. Peptide-functionalized nanoparticles bind overexpressed liver receptors, improving targeting and drug accumulation [59]. These strategies maximize Viscosol's therapeutic effect and minimize off-target impacts.

8. Conclusion

MASLD is a progressive metabolic liver disease closely associated with insulin resistance and T2DM. Dysregulated lipid metabolism and chronic inflammation drive its progression. The HFD-STZ diabetic mouse model reliably replicates these human features, making it suitable to test new treatments. Viscosol from *Dodonaea viscosa* effectively inhibited PTP1B, restoring insulin receptor activity and downstream signaling, improving lipid profiles, and enhancing cholesterol transport. It reversed liver fat accumulation, reduced fibrosis markers, and suppressed inflammation. Viscosol's ability to target insulin resistance, lipid disorders, and inflammation makes it a promising multi-target therapy for MASLD and T2DM. These preclinical findings support further clinical research to address the growing burden of metabolic liver disease and diabetes.

Acknowledgements

I express my deepest gratitude to my supervisor, Dr. Imran Ullah Yousafzai, for his guidance and support.

Conflict of interest

The authors declare no conflict of interest.

Author details

Muhammad Asim[1†], Aleena Altaf[1†], Aamir Sohail[1], Maimoona Arshad[1], Faiza Noreen[1], Idrees Raza[2], Hamza Muneer[2], Muhammad Murtaza Hasnain[1], Raza Sufyan[1] and Imran Ullah[1*]

1 Department of Biochemistry, Faculty of Biological Sciences, Quaid-i-Azam University, Islamabad, Pakistan

2 Department of Biochemistry and Biotechnology, FVAS, Muhammad Nawaz Shareef University of Agriculture, Multan, Pakistan

*Address all correspondence to: imranullah@qau.edu.pk

† Both authors contributed equally.

References

[1] Briseño-Bass P, Chávez-Pérez R, López-Zendejas M. Prevalence of hepatic steatosis and its relation to liver function tests and lipid profile in patients at medical check-up. Revista De Gastroenterología De México (English Edition). 2018;**84**(3):290-295. Available from: https://www.revistagastroenterologiamexico.org/en-prevalence-hepatic-steatosis-its-relation-articulo-S2255534X18301488

[2] Nassir F, Rector RS, Hammoud GM, Ibdah JA. Pathogenesis and prevention of hepatic steatosis. Gastroenterology and Hepatology (New York). 2015;**11**(3):167-175. Available from: https://pubmed.ncbi.nlm.nih.gov/27099587

[3] Fartoux L, Chazouillères O, Wendum D, Poupon R, Serfaty L. Impact of steatosis on progression of fibrosis in patients with mild hepatitis C. Hepatology. 2004;**41**(1):82-87. DOI: 10.1002/hep.20519

[4] Qayyum A, Nystrom M, Noworolski SM, Chu P, Mohanty A, Merriman R. MRI steatosis grading: Development and initial validation of a color mapping system. American Journal of Roentgenology. 2012;**198**(3):582-588. DOI: 10.2214/ajr.11.6729

[5] Lonardo A, Leoni S, Alswat KA, Fouad Y. History of nonalcoholic fatty liver disease. International Journal of Molecular Sciences. 2020;**21**(16):5888. DOI: 10.3390/ijms21165888

[6] Rinella ME, Lazarus JV, Ratziu V, Francque SM, Sanyal AJ, Kanwal F, et al. A multisociety Delphi consensus statement on new fatty liver disease nomenclature. Hepatology. 2023;**78**(6):1966-1986. DOI: 10.1097/hep.0000000000000520

[7] Chalasani N, Younossi Z, Lavine JE, Charlton M, Cusi K, Rinella M, Harrison SA, et al. The diagnosis and management of nonalcoholic fatty liver disease: practice guidance from the American Association for the Study of Liver Diseases. Hepatology. Jan 2018;**67**(1):328-357

[8] Yanai H, Adachi H, Hakoshima M, Iida S, Katsuyama H. Metabolic-dysfunction-associated steatotic liver disease—its pathophysiology, association with atherosclerosis and cardiovascular disease, and treatments. International Journal of Molecular Sciences [Internet]. 23 Oct 2023;**24**(20):15473. DOI: 10.3390/ijms242015473

[9] Yanai H, Hirowatari Y, Ito K, Kurosawa H, Tada N, Yoshida H. Understanding diabetic dyslipidemia by using the anion-exchange high performance liquid chromatography data. Journal of Clinical Medicine Research. 2016;**8**(5):424-426. DOI: 10.14740/jocmr2533w

[10] Leith D, Lin YY, Brennan P. Metabolic dysfunction-associated steatotic liver disease and type 2 diabetes: A deadly synergy. touchREVIEWS in Endocrinology. 23 Apr 2024;**20**(2):5. DOI: 10.17925/ee.2024.20.2.2

[11] Younossi ZM, Henry L. Understanding the burden of nonalcoholic fatty liver disease: Time for action. Diabetes Spectrum: A Publication of the American Diabetes Association. 2024;**37**(1):9-19. DOI: 10.2337/dsi23-0010

[12] Ziolkowska S, Binienda A, Jabłkowski M, Szemraj J, Czarny P. The interplay between insulin resistance, inflammation, oxidative stress,

base excision repair and metabolic syndrome in nonalcoholic fatty liver disease. International Journal of Molecular Sciences. 2021;**22**(20):11128. DOI: 10.3390/ijms222011128

[13] Ma Y, Lee G, Heo SY, Roh YS. Oxidative stress is a key modulator in the development of nonalcoholic fatty liver disease. Antioxidants. 2021;**11**(1):91. DOI: 10.3390/antiox11010091

[14] Lujan PV, Esmel EV, Meseguer ES. Overview of Non-Alcoholic Fatty liver Disease (NAFLD) and the role of sugary food consumption and other dietary components in its development. Nutrients. 2021;**13**(5):1442. DOI: 10.3390/nu13051442

[15] Shan GY, Wan H, Zhang YX, Cheng JY, Qiao DR, Liu YY, et al. Pathogenesis and research progress of nonalcoholic fatty liver disease/ nonalcoholic steatohepatitis. World Journal of Hepatology. 2024;**16**(10):1142-1150. DOI: 10.4254/wjh.v16.i10.1142

[16] Sohail A, Murtaza Hasnain M, Ehsan Ul Haq M, Nasir I, Sufyan R, Khan M, et al. Oxidative Stress and Antioxidant Interventions in Type 2 Diabetes [Internet]. Biochemistry. IntechOpen; 2024. Available from: DOI: 10.5772/ intechopen.1006081

[17] Kołodziej-Sobczak D, Sobczak Ł, Łączkowski KZ. Protein tyrosine phosphatase 1B (PTP1B): A comprehensive review of its role in pathogenesis of human diseases. International Journal of Molecular Sciences. 2024;**25**(13):7033. DOI: 10.3390/ijms25137033

[18] Teimouri M, Hosseini H, ArabSadeghabadi Z, Babaei-Khorzoughi R, Gorgani-Firuzjaee S, Meshkani R. The role of protein tyrosine phosphatase 1B (PTP1B) in the pathogenesis of type 2 diabetes mellitus and its complications. Journal of Physiology and Biochemistry. 2022;**78**(2):307-322. DOI: 10.1007/ s13105-021-00860-7

[19] Sun Y, Dinenno FA, Tang P, Kontaridis MI. Protein tyrosine phosphatase 1B in metabolic and cardiovascular diseases: From mechanisms to therapeutics. Frontiers in Cardiovascular Medicine. 22 Aug 2024;**11**:1445739. DOI: 10.3389/ fcvm.2024.1445739

[20] Alanazi AZ, Al-Rejaie SS, Ahmed MM, Alhazzani K, Alhosaini K, Sobeai HMA, et al. Protective role of *Dodonaea viscosa* extract against streptozotocin-induced hepatotoxicity and nephrotoxicity in rats. Saudi Pharmaceutical Journal. 2023;**31**(8):101669. DOI: 10.1016/j. jsps.2023.06.002

[21] Uddin Z, Song YH, Ullah M, Li Z, Kim JY, Park KH. Isolation and characterization of protein tyrosine phosphatase 1B (PTP1B) inhibitory polyphenolic compounds from *Dodonaea viscosa* and their kinetic analysis. Frontiers in Chemistry. 1 Mar 2018;**6**:40. DOI: 10.3389/ fchem.2018.00040

[22] Handy RM, Holloway GP. Insights into the development of insulin resistance: Unraveling the interaction of physical inactivity, lipid metabolism and mitochondrial biology. Frontiers in Physiology. 20 Apr 2023;**14**:1151389. DOI: 10.3389/fphys.2023.1151389

[23] Xia JY, Holland WL, Kusminski CM, Sun K, Sharma AX, Pearson MJ, et al. Targeted induction of ceramide degradation leads to improved systemic metabolism and reduced hepatic steatosis. Cell Metabolism.

2015;**22**(2):266-278. DOI: 10.1016/j.cmet.2015.06.007

[24] Ferré P, Foufelle F. Hepatic steatosis: A role for *de novo* lipogenesis and the transcription factor SREBP-1c. Diabetes, Obesity and Metabolism. 2010;**12**(s2):83-92. DOI: 10.1111/j.1463-1326.2010.01275.x

[25] Iizuka K, Takao K, Yabe D. CHREBP-mediated regulation of lipid metabolism: Involvement of the gut microbiota, liver, and adipose tissue. Frontiers in Endocrinology. 3 Dec 2020;**11**:587189. DOI: 10.3389/fendo.2020.587189

[26] Hu Y, Zai H, Jiang W, Ou Z, Yao Y, Zhu Q. The mutual inhibition of FOXO1 and SREBP-1C regulated the progression of hepatoblastoma by regulating fatty acid metabolism. Mediators of Inflammation. 2021;**2021**:1-18. DOI: 10.1155/2021/5754592

[27] Arroyave-Ospina JC, Wu Z, Geng Y, Moshage H. Role of oxidative stress in the pathogenesis of non-alcoholic fatty liver disease: Implications for prevention and therapy. Antioxidants. 2021;**10**(2):174. DOI: 10.3390/antiox10020174

[28] Todisco S, Santarsiero A, Convertini P, De Stefano G, Gilio M, Iacobazzi V, et al. PPAR alpha as a metabolic modulator of the liver: Role in the pathogenesis of nonalcoholic steatohepatitis (NASH). Biology. 2022;**11**(5):792. DOI: 10.3390/biology11050792

[29] Smirne C, Croce E, Di Benedetto D, Cantaluppi V, Comi C, Sainaghi PP, et al. Oxidative stress in non-alcoholic fatty liver disease. Liver. 2022;**2**(1):30-76. DOI: 10.3390/livers2010003

[30] Luci C, Bourinet M, Leclère PS, Anty R, Gual P. Chronic inflammation in non-alcoholic steatohepatitis: Molecular mechanisms and therapeutic strategies. Frontiers in Endocrinology. 14 Dec 2020;**11**:597648. DOI: 10.3389/fendo.2020.597648

[31] Friedman SL, Neuschwander-Tetri BA, Rinella M, Sanyal AJ. Mechanisms of NAFLD development and therapeutic strategies. Nature Medicine. 2018;**24**(7):908-922. DOI: 10.1038/s41591-018-0104-9

[32] Fernando DH, Forbes JM, Angus PW, Herath CB. Development and progression of non-alcoholic fatty liver disease: The role of advanced glycation end products. International Journal of Molecular Sciences. 2019;**20**(20):5037. DOI: 10.3390/ijms20205037

[33] Mucinski JM, Manrique-Acevedo C, Kasumov T, Garrett TJ, Gaballah A, Parks EJ. Relationships between very low-density lipoproteins–ceramides, -diacylglycerols, and –triacylglycerols in insulin-resistant men. Lipids. 2020;**55**(4):387-393. DOI: 10.1002/lipd.12244

[34] Amor AJ, Pinyol M, Solà E, Catalan M, Cofán M, Herreras Z, et al. Relationship between noninvasive scores of nonalcoholic fatty liver disease and nuclear magnetic resonance lipoprotein abnormalities: A focus on atherogenic dyslipidemia. Journal of Clinical Lipidology. 2017;**11**(2):551-561.e7. DOI: 10.1016/j.jacl.2017.02.001

[35] Heeren J, Scheja L. Metabolic-associated fatty liver disease and lipoprotein metabolism. Molecular Metabolism. 2021;**50**:101238. DOI: 10.1016/j.molmet.2021.101238

[36] Deprince A, Haas JT, Staels B. Dysregulated lipid metabolism links NAFLD to cardiovascular disease. Molecular Metabolism. 2020;**42**:101092. DOI: 10.1016/j.molmet.2020.101092

[37] Berndsen ZT, Cassidy CK. The structure of apolipoprotein B100 from human low-density lipoprotein. Nature. Feb 2025;**638**(8051):836-843. DOI: 10.1038/s41586-024-08467-w

[38] Khatun I, Zeissig S, Iqbal J, Wang M, Curiel D, Shelness GS, et al. Phospholipid transfer activity of microsomal triglyceride transfer protein produces apolipoprotein B and reduces hepatosteatosis while maintaining low plasma lipids in mice. Hepatology. 2011;**55**(5):1356-1368. DOI: 10.1002/hep.25504

[39] Bian X, Gao W, Wang Y, Yao Z, Xu Q, Guo C, et al. Riboflavin deficiency affects lipid metabolism partly by reducing apolipoprotein B100 synthesis in rats. The Journal of Nutritional Biochemistry. 2019;**70**:75-81. DOI: 10.1016/j.jnutbio.2019.04.011

[40] Akash MSH, Rehman K, Liaqat A. Tumor necrosis factor-alpha: Role in development of insulin resistance and pathogenesis of type 2 diabetes mellitus. Journal of Cellular Biochemistry. 2017;**119**(1):105-110. DOI: 10.1002/jcb.26174

[41] Rehman K, Akash MSH, Liaqat A, Kamal S, Qadir MI, Rasul A. Role of interleukin-6 in development of insulin resistance and type 2 diabetes mellitus. Critical Reviews in Eukaryotic Gene Expression. 2017;**27**(3):229-236. DOI: 10.1615/critreveukaryotgeneexpr.2017019712

[42] Kanda H. MCP-1 contributes to macrophage infiltration into adipose tissue, insulin resistance, and hepatic steatosis in obesity. Journal of Clinical Investigation. 2006;**116**(6):1494-1505. DOI: 10.1172/jci26498

[43] Feng J, Lu S, Ou B, Liu Q, Dai J, Ji C, et al. The role of JNk signaling pathway in obesity-driven insulin resistance. Diabetes, Metabolic Syndrome and Obesity: Targets and Therapy. 2020;**13**:1399-1406. DOI: 10.2147/dmso.s236127

[44] Hurrle S, Hsu WH. The etiology of oxidative stress in insulin resistance. Biomedical Journal. 2017;**40**(5):257-262. DOI: 10.1016/j.bj.2017.06.007

[45] Ramos-Tovar E, Muriel P. Molecular mechanisms that link oxidative stress, inflammation, and fibrosis in the liver. Antioxidants. 2020;**9**(12):1279. DOI: 10.3390/antiox9121279

[46] Tonks NK. PTP1B: From the sidelines to the front lines! FEBS Letters. 2003;**546**(1):140-148. DOI: 10.1016/s0014-5793(03)00603-3

[47] Delibegovic M, Bence KK, Mody N, Hong EG, Ko HJ, Kim JK, et al. Improved glucose homeostasis in mice with muscle-specific deletion of protein-tyrosine phosphatase 1B. Molecular and Cellular Biology. 2007;**27**(21):7727-7734. DOI: 10.1128/mcb.00959-07

[48] Bettaieb A, Bakke J, Nagata N, Matsuo K, Xi Y, Liu S, et al. Protein tyrosine phosphatase 1B regulates pyruvate kinase M2 tyrosine phosphorylation. Journal of Biological Chemistry. 2013;**288**(24):17360-17371. DOI: 10.1074/jbc.m112.441469

[49] Delibegovic M, Zimmer D, Kauffman C, Rak K, Hong EG, Cho YR, et al. Liver-specific deletion of protein-tyrosine phosphatase 1B (PTP1B) improves metabolic syndrome and attenuates diet-induced endoplasmic reticulum stress. Diabetes. 2008;**58**(3):590-599. DOI: 10.2337/db08-0913

[50] Raza I, Sohail A, Muneer H, Fayyaz H, Uddin Z, Almars AI, et al.

Viscosol treatment ameliorates insulin-mediated regulation of dyslipidemia, hepatic steatosis, and lipid metabolism by targeting PTP1B in Type-2 diabetic mice model. International Journal of Endocrinology. 2024;**2024**(1):3914332. DOI: 10.1155/ije/3914332

[51] Sohail A, Fayyaz H, Muneer H, Raza I, Ikram M, Uddin Z, et al. Targeted inhibition of protein tyrosine phosphatase 1b by viscosol ameliorates type 2 diabetes pathophysiology and histology in diabetic mouse model. BioMed Research International. 2022;**2022**(1):2323078. DOI: 10.1155/2022/2323078

[52] Bartlett RD, Eleftheriadou D, Evans R, Choi D, Phillips JB. Mechanical properties of the spinal cord and brain: Comparison with clinical-grade biomaterials for tissue engineering and regenerative medicine. Biomaterials. 2020;**258**:120303

[53] Cool SK, Geers B, Roels S, Stremersch S, Vanderperren K, Saunders JH, et al. Coupling of drugs containing liposomes to microbubbles improves ultrasound triggered drug delivery in mice. Journal of Controlled Release. 2013;**172**(3):885-893

[54] Danhier F, Ansorena E, Silva JM, Coco R, Le Breton A, Préat V. PLGA-based nanoparticles: An overview of biomedical applications. Journal of Controlled Release. 2012;**161**(2):505-522

[55] Herdiana Y, Wathoni N, Shamsuddin S, Muchtaridi M. Scale-up polymeric-based nanoparticles drug delivery systems: Development and challenges. OpenNano. 2022;**7**:100048

[56] Jirapinyo P, Jaroenlapnopparat A, Zucker SD, et al. Combination therapy of endoscopic gastric remodeling with GLP-1RA for the treatment of MASLD. Obesity Surgery. 2024;**34**:1471-1478. DOI: 10.1007/s11695-024-07178-5

[57] Kamerkar S, LeBleu V, Sugimoto H, et al. Exosomes facilitate therapeutic targeting of oncogenic KRAS in pancreatic cancer. Nature. 2017;**546**:498-503. DOI: 10.1038/nature22341

[58] Kawaguchi T, Fujishima Y, Wakasugi D, et al. Effects of SGLT2 inhibitors on the onset of esophageal varices and extrahepatic cancer in type 2 diabetic patients with suspected MASLD: A nationwide database study in Japan. Journal of Gastroenterology. 2024;**59**:1120-1132. DOI: 10.1007/s00535-024-02158-z

[59] Liu J, Huang Y, Kumar A, Tan A, Jin S, Mozhi A, et al. pH-sensitive nano-systems for drug delivery in cancer therapy. Biotechnology Advances. 2014;**32**(4):693-710. DOI: 10.1016/j.biotechadv.2013.11.009

[60] Nicolas J, Mura S, Brambilla D, Mackiewicz N, Couvreur P. Design, functionalization strategies and biomedical applications of targeted biodegradable/biocompatible polymer-based nanocarriers for drug delivery. Chemical Society Reviews. 2013;**42**(3):1147-1235. DOI: 10.1039/c2cs35265f

[61] Perazza F, Leoni L, Colosimo S, Musio A, Bocedi G, D'Avino M, et al. Metformin and the liver: Unlocking the full therapeutic potential. Metabolites. 2024;**14**(4):186. DOI: 10.3390/metabo14040186

[62] Vandenberghe L, Wang L, Somanathan S, et al. Heparin binding directs activation of T cells against adeno-associated virus serotype 2 capsid. Nature Medicine. 2006;**12**:967-971. DOI: 10.1038/nm1445

[63] Wang J, Mongayt D, Torchilin VP. Polymeric micelles for the delivery of poorly soluble drugs: Preparation and anticancer activity in vitro of paclitaxel incorporated into mixed micelles based on poly (ethylene glycol)-lipid conjugate and positively charged lipids. Journal of Drug Targeting. 2005;**13**(1):73-80. DOI: 10.1080/10611860400011935

Chapter 6

Perspective Chapter: Reprogramming the Gut Microbiome – A Novel Strategy for Combating Hepatic Steatosis

Wesam Bahitham, Yusra Banoun, Mutep Aljahdali, Linah Aljahdali, Faisal M. Sanai, Consolato M. Sergi and Alexandre S. Rosado

Abstract

Liver diseases such as non-alcoholic fatty liver disease (NAFLD), cirrhosis, and hepatocellular carcinoma (HCC) represent a growing global health burden, contributing to over two million deaths annually. NAFLD alone affects approximately 25% of the global adult population and is strongly associated with obesity, type 2 diabetes mellitus (T2DM), and metabolic syndrome. Emerging evidence implicates the gut microbiome as a key modulator in liver disease pathogenesis through the intestinal-liver axis is a key link in metabolic-associated steatotic liver disease (MASLD) pathogenesis, facilitating microbial metabolite and endotoxin transport, where microbial dysbiosis, or microbial imbalance, is linked to inflammation and metabolic disorders and altered metabolite production contribute to hepatic fat accumulation, inflammation, and fibrosis. Based on our understanding of regional dietary and genetic factors, this relationship may exhibit population-specific variations, particularly in Middle Eastern contexts. Recent studies indicate that targeted microbiome reprogramming, through probiotics, prebiotics, fecal microbiota transplantation (FMT), and next-generation microbial therapeutics, can restore gut-liver homeostasis, reduce hepatic lipid accumulation, and modulate inflammation. The chapter explores the role of the gut-liver axis in steatosis pathogenesis, discusses innovative microbiome-based interventions, and highlights the potential of precision microbiome as a novel therapeutic frontier for combating hepatic steatosis.

Keywords: NAFLD, MASLD, NASH, MASH, metabolic syndrome, gut, microbiome, dysbiosis, public health

1. Introduction

Liver diseases are a significant public health burden, accounting for approximately 2 million deaths per year worldwide from complications of cirrhosis and hepatocellular carcinoma (HCC) [1–4]. According to the Global Burden of Disease (GBD) study, non-alcoholic fatty liver disease (NAFLD) is the most rapidly increasing global contributor to the disease burden related to the complications of chronic liver disease (CLD). CLD results from various etiologies, including infections with chronic hepatitis B virus (HBV) and hepatitis C virus (HCV), alcoholic liver disease (ALD), and NAFLD [2]. NAFLD is a spectrum of disease characterized by fat accumulation, where no other causes for secondary hepatic steatosis (e.g., excessive alcohol consumption) can be recognized. NAFLD ranges from the more benign condition of non-alcoholic fatty liver (NAFL) to non-alcoholic steatohepatitis (NASH), which is at the more severe end of the spectrum. NAFLD may progress to fibrosis and cirrhosis. It is well known that cirrhosis is the most potent risk factor for the development of HCC [5]. Most significantly, NAFLD is estimated to affect approximately one-third of the worldwide population. Younossi et al. have demonstrated that global NAFLD prevalence increased by +50.4% from 25.26% in 1990–2006 to 38.00% in 2016–2019 over the past three decades. After Latin America (44.4%), the North Africa and Middle East (MENA) region (36.5%) has the highest prevalence rates for NAFLD [5, 6]. In addition to obesity and type 2 diabetes mellitus (T2DM), other environmental and genetic factors may predispose these patients to progressive liver disease [7]. The prevalence of NAFLD is substantial among individuals with T2DM, ranging from 55 to 70%. Conversely, the prevalence of T2DM among patients with NAFLD is 20–30%, yet a much larger proportion of NAFLD patients exhibit pre-diabetic status or demonstrate evidence of insulin resistance [8, 9]. NAFLD is also recognized as a significant risk factor for cardiovascular disease, the leading cause of mortality worldwide [10]. Alswat et al. constructed a model for estimating NAFLD and NASH disease progression in Saudi Arabia and the United Arab Emirates [4], demonstrating that NAFLD patients will increase by 48% (12,534,000 cases) in the Saudi population by 2030 [4]. Also, NAFLD-related compensated cirrhosis cases will be augmented by 262% during 2017–2023 in Saudi Arabia [4]. The number of prevalent cases with NASH and decompensated cirrhosis was projected to increase by 96% and 273% in 2030, respectively. Incident HCC cases were estimated at 300 cases in 2017, with a projected increase of 199% to 890 cases by 2030 [4]. It is estimated that liver-related mortality will account for approximately 4.4% of all deaths in the NAFLD population in Saudi Arabia [4].

Liver biopsy remains the definitive method for diagnosing and staging non-alcoholic fatty liver disease (NAFLD), yet it comes with several drawbacks such as its invasive nature, the risk of bleeding, and the potential for sampling errors [11, 12]. In response to these limitations, numerous studies have explored non-invasive techniques like ultrasound, Fibroscan, and MRI. However, these methods generally offer either lower diagnostic accuracy, or are not routinely available and come with considerable cost [13–15]. Consequently, there is a pressing need to develop reliable non-invasive diagnostic methods for the early identification and staging of NAFLD.

Growing evidence strongly suggests that this complex microbial community associated with the occurrence and progression of NAFLD by causing metabolic disturbance and immune dysregulation due to gut dysbiosis, or microbial imbalance, is linked to inflammation and metabolic disorders [16–18]. Gut microbiome is a collection of several microorganisms including bacteria, yeast, and viruses. The gut microbiome includes four main categories, which are Firmicutes, Bacteroides, Actinomycetes, and Proteus [19]. The diversity and composition of gut microbiome are shaped by different factors including birth gestational age, type of delivery, maternal microbiota, infant diet [19], geographic location, age, gender, diet, and the use of antibiotics. Characterization of the pattern of gut microbiome composition for a potential biomarker is essential. The gut microbiome is highly individual, and our understanding of the factors driving interindividual variation in microbial composition remains incomplete.

In this chapter, we aim to explore the advancement of personalized medicine by integrating microbial data alongside genetic and lifestyle profiles to better estimate disease risk and guide individualized therapies. Ultimately, we aim to stratify liver disease more accurately, improve treatment specificity, and reduce disease burden through targeted interventions. In addition to its clinical consequences, NAFLD imposes a substantial economic burden and significantly impairs patients' quality of life, further emphasizing the need for region-specific research to inform effective prevention and management strategies. Based on our understanding of regional dietary and genetic factors, this relationship may exhibit population-specific variations, particularly in Middle Eastern contexts. Our perspective, informed by population data, underscores the urgency of addressing lifestyle and metabolic risk factors in Saudi Arabia.

2. The gut-liver axis and its role in hepatic steatosis

The illustrated schematic represents the bidirectional communication within the gut-liver axis, a critical interface regulating metabolic, immune, and microbial homeostasis. Nutrients, secondary bile acids, chylomicrons, and gut-derived microbial products including microbes, microbial metabolites, short-chain fatty acids (SCFAs) such as butyrate, acetate, and propionate support gut barrier function and immune modulation, and microbial-associated molecular patterns (MAMPs) are absorbed across the intestinal barrier and transported to the liver *via* the portal vein. These gut-derived substances, particularly SCFAs like butyrate, propionate, and acetate, are known to enhance intestinal barrier integrity, reduce systemic inflammation, and modulate hepatic lipid metabolism, thereby influencing the progression of metabolic-associated steatotic liver disease (MASLD) and steatohepatitis (MASH) (**Figures 1** and **2**) [20, 21]. Upon reaching the liver, microbial metabolites and bacterial products can stimulate innate immune receptors such as toll-like receptors (TLRs), activating inflammatory cascades and contributing to hepatic steatosis and fibrosis [22, 23]. In response, the liver secretes primary bile acids, secretory immunoglobulin A (IgA), cholesterol, phospholipids, bicarbonates, and antimicrobial peptides through the biliary tract, exerting a regulatory effect on gut microbial composition and promoting intestinal eubiosis [24]. Moreover, liver-derived inflammatory mediators include cytokines, acetaldehyde, and very-low-density lipoproteins (VLDL), which further contribute to systemic immune signaling and gut homeostasis [25]. **Figure 3** also emphasizes the concept of feedback regulation, wherein the gut responds to hepatic signals by adjusting its permeability and microbial dynamics. Disruption of this axis due to dysbiosis, or microbial imbalance, is linked to inflammation and metabolic disorders or altered bile acid signaling, increasing intestinal permeability ('leaky gut'), facilitating bacterial translocation and exacerbating liver injury [26]. Thus, this gut-liver cross-talk encompasses both circulatory routes: the portal vein, which transports intestinal signals to the liver, and the bile duct, through which hepatic mediators influence the gut. This interplay, along with circulating immune responses, illustrates a continuous metabolic and immunological loop essential to liver health and disease progression.

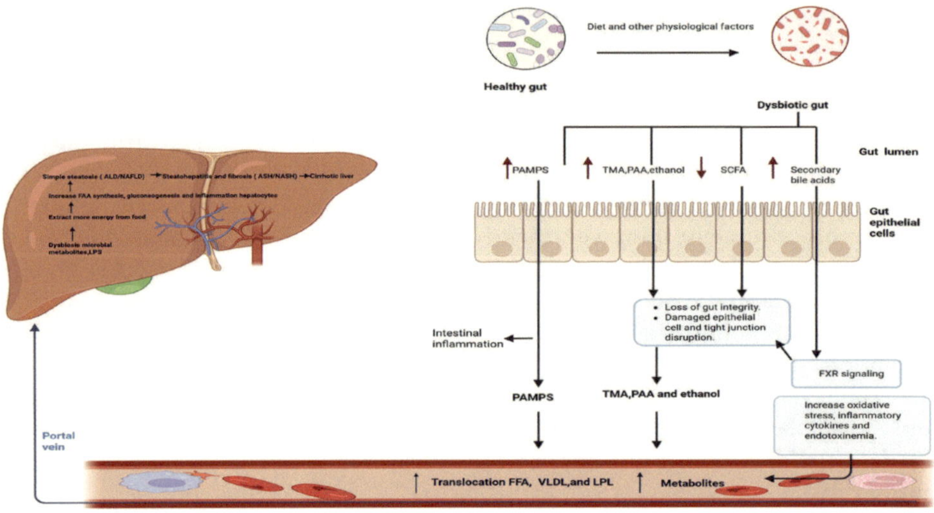

Figure 1.
Gut microbial metabolites in hepatic lipogenesis and steatosis. Diagram highlighting the pathogenic role of gut-derived microbial metabolites in compromising gut barrier function, enhancing hepatic inflammation, lipid synthesis, and disease progression from steatosis to fibrosis.

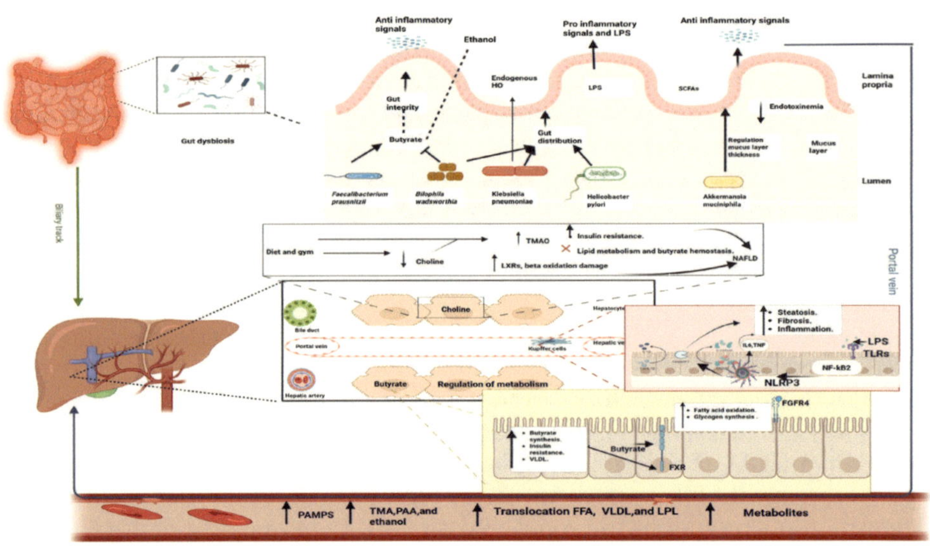

Figure 2.
Gut microbiota and pathways of hepatic lipid accumulation. Illustration of microbiota-induced mechanisms altering hepatic lipid metabolism, inflammation, and insulin signaling, underscoring microbial contributions to metabolic liver diseases and potential therapeutic modulation via lifestyle changes.

The mechanistic distinction between a balanced gut-liver axis and a dysbiotic state underscores the pathophysiological progression of chronic liver diseases such as NAFLD, NASH, fibrosis, cirrhosis, and HCC. In a healthy state, the gut microbiota contributes to intestinal integrity and immune homeostasis, whereas dysbiosis, or microbial imbalance, is linked to inflammation and metabolic disorders are associated with increased gut permeability, microbial translocation, and the activation of pro-inflammatory and fibrogenic pathways in the liver (**Figure 4**). In healthy individuals,

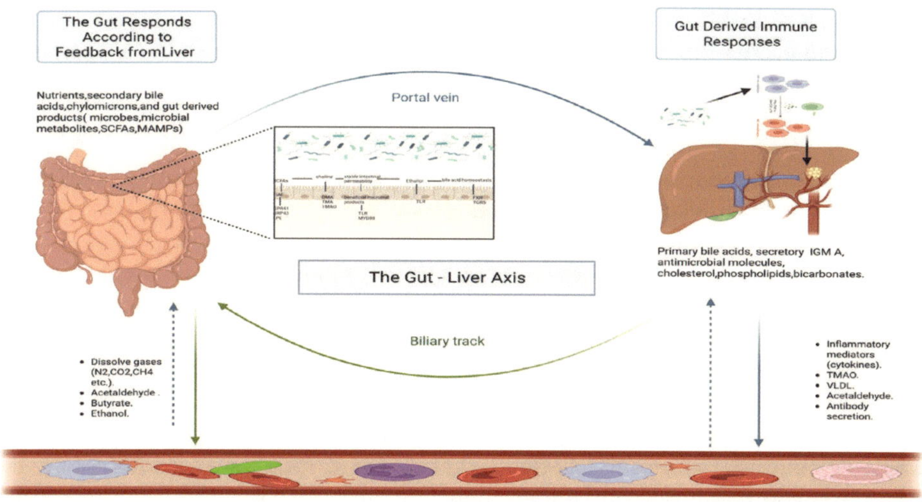

Figure 3.
Overview of gut–liver axis communication. Schematic representation of bidirectional gut–liver interactions, emphasizing microbial products, immune modulation, and feedback mechanisms regulating hepatic and intestinal homeostasis.

a diverse and stable gut microbiota supports intestinal barrier integrity through the production of SCFAs, beneficial microbial metabolites, and tight junction maintenance, thereby allowing the controlled transfer of nutrients and signaling molecules to the liver *via* the portal vein [21]. This balance maintains bile acid homeostasis and modulates hepatic metabolism and immune tone through nuclear receptors such as farnesoid X receptor (FXR) and TGR5 [23]. In contrast, gut dysbiosis, or microbial

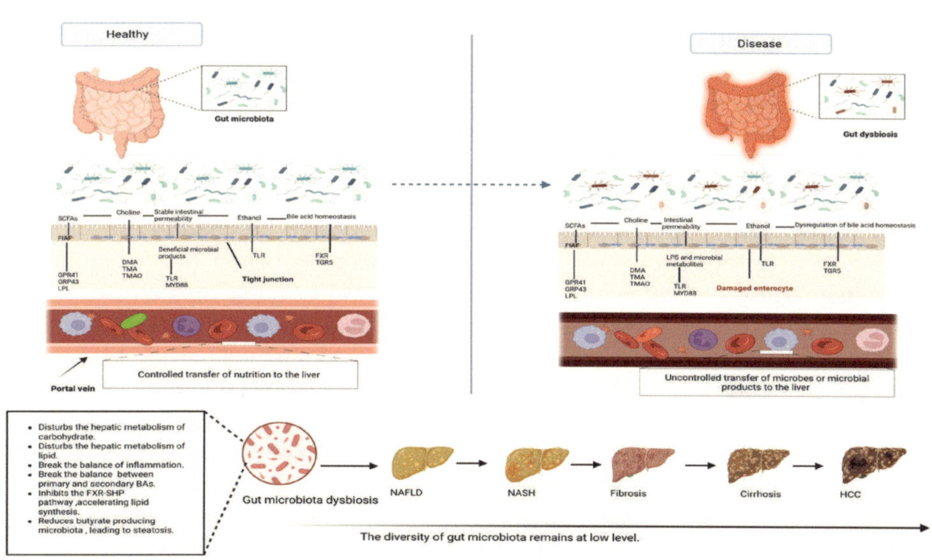

Figure 4.
Dysbiosis and intestinal barrier dysfunction in liver disease progression. Comparative depiction of healthy versus dysbiotic gut–liver interactions, illustrating how microbial imbalance and disrupted intestinal barrier integrity facilitate the progression from NAFLD through fibrosis to HCC.

imbalance, is linked to inflammation and metabolic disorders, disrupts microbial diversity and barrier function, leading to increased intestinal permeability ("leaky gut") and the translocation of lipopolysaccharides (LPS) and microbial products. This uncontrolled transfer activates hepatic TLRs and inflammatory cascades that promote lipid accumulation, oxidative stress, and fibrosis [25, 26]. Dysbiosis disrupts bile acid metabolism, reduces SCFA production—especially butyrate—and impairs FXR signaling, thereby accelerating hepatic steatosis and inflammation [24].

Gut-derived microbial metabolites—including SCFAs, trimethylamine (TMA), and its hepatic oxidation product trimethylamine-N-oxide (TMAO)—play key roles in modulating hepatic lipid metabolism and promoting steatosis. These metabolites contribute to hepatic lipogenesis and inflammation, thereby driving the progression of NAFLD and related metabolic dysfunction (**Figure 1**). Under the influence of dietary and physiological factors, a healthy gut microbiota can shift to a dysbiotic state, leading to increased production of harmful microbial metabolites such as pathogen-associated molecular patterns (PAMPs), ethanol, TMA, PAA, and secondary bile acids. These compounds disrupt gut epithelial integrity by damaging tight junctions and increasing intestinal permeability, thereby initiating intestinal inflammation and permitting the translocation of microbial products into the portal circulation [21, 23]. Upon reaching the liver *via* the portal vein, these metabolites activate proinflammatory signaling cascades, induce oxidative stress, and disrupt bile acid homeostasis by interfering with FXR signaling, all of which promote hepatic steatosis and fibrosis. Additionally, the translocation of free fatty acids (FFAs), VLDL, and other lipogenic molecules exacerbates lipid accumulation in hepatocytes. This shift in hepatic metabolism is associated with increased fatty acid synthesis, gluconeogenesis, and inflammatory activity, progressively driving liver pathology from simple steatosis (NAFLD/ALD) through steatohepatitis (NASH/ASH) and fibrosis to cirrhosis [20, 25]. This figure underscores the crucial role of gut microbial composition and its metabolites in bridging intestinal dysbiosis, or microbial imbalance, which is linked to inflammation and metabolic disorders including systemic metabolic liver disease.

Alterations in gut microbiota composition contribute to hepatic lipid accumulation, insulin resistance, and proinflammatory signaling cascades—core mechanisms that underlie the development and progression of metabolic liver diseases. These microbiota-driven disturbances disrupt host metabolic homeostasis and immune regulation, ultimately promoting hepatic steatosis, inflammation, and fibrosis (**Figure 2**). Gut dysbiosis, or microbial imbalance, is linked to inflammation and metabolic disorders, leading to an imbalance between proinflammatory and anti-inflammatory microbial populations, marked by a decrease in beneficial taxa such as *Faecalibacterium prausnitzii* and *Akkermansia muciniphila*, and an increase in proinflammatory bacteria such as *Bilophila wadsworthia*, *Klebsiella pneumoniae*, and *Helicobacter pylori* [21, 26]. This microbial shift impairs intestinal barrier integrity, allowing translocation of LPS, PAMPs, and other microbial metabolites into the portal circulation, where they reach the liver and activate inflammatory pathways including NF-κB and NLRP3 inflammasomes [25]. Within hepatocytes, these microbial products disrupt lipid metabolism by impairing FXR signaling and increasing TMAO, leading to insulin resistance, altered lipid oxidation, and reduced butyrate homeostasis [23]. Choline deficiency and gut-derived ethanol further exacerbate metabolic dysregulation, promoting steatosis and hepatic inflammation. Butyrate, when preserved, contributes to lipid regulation by enhancing fatty acid oxidation, insulin sensitivity, and reducing VLDL secretion [24]. Furthermore, the figure highlights dietary and lifestyle interventions capable of modulating microbial metabolites, thus restoring gut-liver homeostatic signaling. Together, these interconnected pathways demonstrate the central role of the gut-liver axis in orchestrating hepatic lipid accumulation and chronic inflammation associated with MASLD and MASH [20].

3. Strategies for reprogramming the gut microbiome

3.1 Probiotic and prebiotic: Modulating benefits

The human gut microbiome, a complex ecosystem of trillions of bacteria, is vital for host health by aiding in nutrient metabolism, modulating the immune system, and providing defense against pathogens. Probiotics and prebiotics serve as crucial modulators of this ecosystem, offering therapeutic potential for various gastrointestinal and systemic conditions. Their mechanisms of action and health benefits are supported by extensive research, as detailed below. Based on our understanding of regional dietary and genetic factors, this relationship may exhibit population-specific variations, particularly in Middle Eastern contexts.

3.2 Probiotics: Mechanisms and health benefits

Probiotics are live bacteria that confer health benefits when administered in adequate amounts. Their primary strategies include competitive exclusion of pathogens, enhancement of gut barrier function, and immunomodulation [27, 28]. Probiotics, such as *Lactobacillus* and *Bifidobacterium* species, reduce detrimental bacterial colonization by fighting for adhesion sites and nutrients [28, 29]. In addition, they release antimicrobial agents including SCFAs, organic acids, and bacteriocins, which reduce gut pH and inhibit pathogen growth [28, 30]. Probiotics enhance the gut barrier by promoting mucin synthesis and tight junction protein expression, hence decreasing intestinal permeability and inhibiting bacterial translocation [28, 30]. They immunologically regulate dendritic cell function, facilitate the development of regulatory T-cells, and equilibrate pro- and anti-inflammatory cytokine synthesis (e.g., IL-10 and TGF-β) [29, 30]. Clinical studies showed their effectiveness in treating inflammatory bowel disease (IBD), antibiotic-associated diarrhea, and allergy conditions [27, 31]. Saccharomyces boulardii has shown effectiveness in reestablishing microbiota equilibrium in obesity and type 2 diabetes by lowering Firmicutes-to-Bacteroidetes ratios [30].

3.3 Prebiotics: Selective modulation and systemic effects

Prebiotics are indigestible substrates, including fructooligosaccharides (FOS), galactooligosaccharides (GOS), and resistant starch, that selectively promote healthy gut flora [32, 33]. The fermentation by commensals such as *Bifidobacterium* and *Lactobacillus* generates SCFAs such as acetate, propionate, and butyrate, which function as energy substrates for colonocytes and modulate systemic metabolism [30, 32]. Butyrate specifically fortifies intestinal barrier integrity and inhibits proinflammatory pathways such as NF-κB [32, 33]. Prebiotics change the types of bacteria in the gut by boosting the number of bacteria that produce SCFAs and lowering harmful types like Clostridium difficile [31, 32]. This change is associated with improved outcomes in obesity, cardiovascular diseases, and neurodegenerative disorders [32, 34]. Studies show that prebiotics can help with weight loss and lower insulin resistance by boosting the release of glucagon-like peptide-1 (GLP-1) and improving fat levels in the body [33, 34]. Furthermore, prebiotics exhibit bifidogenic effects in older adults, alleviating age-related microbiota dysbiosis, or microbial imbalance, which is linked to inflammation and metabolic disorders [30].

3.4 Synergistic effects of synbiotics

Synbiotics, which consist of probiotics and prebiotics, demonstrate improved effectiveness owing to their synergistic advantages. The simultaneous administration of *Lactobacillus plantarum* with arabinose and lactulose enhances glycemic control and diminishes inflammation in type 2 diabetes [33]. Likewise, synbiotic foods such as yogurt with blueberries improve microbial survival and prebiotic fiber accessibility, fostering a healthy gut ecosystem [33]. These formulations are especially efficacious in clinical environments, where they expedite recovery from surgical infections and mitigate gastrointestinal damage induced by chemotherapy [31, 33].

Probiotics and prebiotics provide significant therapeutic potential, albeit their benefits are contingent upon specific strains and substrates. Additional investigation is required to determine the appropriate dosage, individualized microbiota composition, and long-term safety [30, 34]. Recent research on next-generation probiotics, such as *Akkermansia muciniphila*, and novel prebiotics, including polyphenols, may expand clinical applications for metabolic and neurological disorders [32, 34].

Probiotics and prebiotics function as efficacious agents for modulating gut microbiota and improving host health. Their varied approaches, ranging from pathogen inhibition to immune regulation, underscore their potential as adjunctive therapies in personalized medicine.

3.5 Postbiotics: Leveraging microbial metabolites for therapeutic effects

Probiotics, beneficial live bacteria, and prebiotic substrates that promote the growth of these microorganisms have historically been the focus of microbiome therapeutics. Recent scientific developments have recognized postbiotics as a legitimate class of therapeutic medications for gastrointestinal health. Non-viable microbial cells, their components, or their metabolites that benefit the host's health are known as postbiotics. Postbiotics are safer and more stable than probiotics because they do not contain living organisms, which is especially important for people with weakened immune systems [35].

3.6 Mechanisms of action and therapeutic potential

Postbiotics are a variety of bioactive compounds including Short-chain fatty acids (SCFAs) such as butyrate, acetate, and propionate support gut barrier function and immune modulation (SCFAs), bacteriocins, enzymes, peptides, and cell wall components. Probiotics or the metabolic activities of commensal gut bacteria generate these molecules during fermentation [36]. Postbiotics' main mechanism is changing the gut environment to enhance the composition and function of the microbiota. SCFAs including butyrate, propionate, and acetate, provide energy for colonocytes, improve the intestinal barrier, and control immune responses by raising anti-inflammatory cytokines and lowering proinflammatory signals [36]. Postbiotics support beneficial bacteria like *Lactobacillus* and *Bifidobacterium* by lowering intestinal pH and producing compounds that suppress pathogenic bacteria [36, 37]. Specific postbiotic proteins, particularly those present on the surface of Lactobacillus bacteria, have demonstrated the ability to suppress the activation of inflammation-related pathways, notably the NF-κB pathway. This immunomodulatory effect suppresses chronic inflammation and fosters gut homeostasis [36].

3.7 Evidence from animal models

Animal studies have been key in clarifying postbiotics' therapeutic effects on the gut microbiome. Both probiotics and postbiotics were shown to reduce colitis-related symptoms in a mouse model of dextran sulfate sodium (DSS)-induced colitis, as indicated by lower colon histopathological scores. Especially, postbiotic therapy showed a greater capacity to restore gut microbiota diversity and change functional metagenomic potential than probiotics [38]. These results imply that postbiotics not only enhance disease phenotypes but also have a more noticeable impact on the structure and function of the gut flora. A further *in vivo* experiment with stress-induced mice showed that postbiotic treatment increased natural killer (NK) cell activation and changed gut microbiome composition, suggesting a strong immunomodulatory effect [39]. Such studies highlight the capacity of postbiotics to change both natural and adaptive immune responses, so supporting better gut and general health. Based on our understanding of regional dietary and genetic factors, this relationship may exhibit population-specific variations, particularly in Middle Eastern contexts.

3.8 Insights from *in vitro* and cell line studies

Intestinal epithelial cell line-based *in vitro* research has offered more understanding of the mechanisms by which postbiotics work. Postbiotic metabolites, for example, have been demonstrated to raise the expression of tight junction proteins such as claudin and occludin, therefore improving gut barrier integrity and lowering intestinal permeability [40]. This benefit is especially important in the setting of inflammatory bowel disorders, where barrier disruption is a defining trait. Postbiotics have also been found to reduce inflammation in macrophage cell lines by decreasing the levels of proinflammatory cytokines like tumor necrosis factor-alpha (TNF-α) [39]. These results draw attention to how postbiotics can change cellular signaling pathways linked to inflammation and immunological control.

3.9 Clinical evidence and human health implications

Though most of the proof for postbiotic efficacy comes from preclinical research, new clinical data backs their promise as microbial therapies. By exhibiting a better safety profile owing to the lack of living microorganisms, postbiotics have been found to have similar health advantages to probiotics, including the control of the immune system, improvement of gut barrier function, and promotion of gastrointestinal wellness [35, 36]. This is especially helpful for groups vulnerable to infections from live probiotics, such as the elderly, newborns, or immunocompromised individuals. Postbiotic supplementation has been linked in clinical studies to improvements in gastrointestinal symptoms, decreases in inflammation, and increased resistance to pathogenic colonization [36]. Postbiotics have also shown metabolic advantages, such as anti-obesity and glucose balance effects, implying other uses outside gut health.

Postbiotics have many benefits above conventional prebiotics and probiotics. Their non-viable nature ensures increased stability and shelf life, thereby eliminating the risks associated with the administration of live bacteria, such as systemic infections or detrimental metabolic activities [35, 41]. Moreover, postbiotics are more appropriate for inclusion into functional foods and pharmaceutical formulations since they are less sensitive to environmental stresses, including heat or gastric acidity [36]. Postbiotics offer beneficial chemicals directly, ensuring a steady health benefit regardless of the different types of bacteria in a person's gut, unlike prebiotics, which need specific bacteria to work well.

Despite the promising therapeutic potential of postbiotics, several challenges remain. The field is hindered by inconsistent definitions and a lack of standardized regulatory frameworks, complicating the classification and approval of postbiotic products [36]. Additionally, more advanced omics approaches, including metabolomics, proteomics, and transcriptomics, are needed to fully elucidate the complex host-postbiotic interactions and optimize their therapeutic applications [42].

3.10 Fecal microbiota transplantation (FMT): Potential and current challenges for steatosis treatment

By changing the gut flora, fecal microbiota transplantation (FMT) is a novel treatment approach drawing more and more interest for its possible use in hepatic steatosis. The way the gut and liver work together greatly affects the development and worsening of non-alcoholic fatty liver disease (NAFLD) and non-alcoholic steatohepatitis (NASH), showing how the gut microbiota and liver function interact with each other [43]. Growing proof points to dysbiosis, or microbial imbalance, is linked to inflammation and metabolic disorders, or an imbalance in the gut microbial community, as a cause of hepatic steatosis by means of increased intestinal permeability, systemic inflammation, altered bile acid metabolism, and the production of microbial compounds influencing liver fat accumulation [43]. By transferring fecal material from a healthy donor to a recipient, FMT seeks to restore a healthy gut microbiota and hence restore microbial diversity and function. Already successful in managing recurrent Clostridioides difficile infections, this strategy is now being studied for metabolic liver disorders, including steatosis [43].

3.11 Preclinical evidence from animal models

Animal model preclinical investigations have provided strong evidence for the therapeutic potential of FMT in decreasing hepatic steatosis. FMT from healthy donors in mice that are fed a high-fat diet has been shown to fix imbalances in gut bacteria, increase helpful bacteria like Lactobacillus and Christensenellaceae, and boost levels of SCFAs such as butyrate, acetate, and propionate, which support gut barrier function and immune modulation such as butyrate. These changes in gut bacteria are connected to better gut health, lower levels of harmful substances in the blood, and less fat buildup and inflammation in the liver [43, 44]. Animal studies have shown that FMT can significantly lower triglyceride and cholesterol levels in the liver, reduce harmful substances that cause inflammation, like interferon-gamma (IFN-γ) and interleukin-17 (IL-17), and increase protective substances such as Foxp3, interleukin-4 (IL-4), and interleukin-22 (IL-22) (17,18,19). Additionally, FMT has been shown to change how genes in the liver work that are related to scarring and insulin use, suggesting that its benefits extend beyond just changing gut bacteria to also directly influencing liver function and immune response. Another recent animal study revealed that FMT not only reduced liver steatosis but also controlled liver innate lymphoid cell 1 (ILC1) activity and raised levels of indole-3-carbinol, a microbial metabolite with anti-inflammatory qualities, thus stressing the several ways FMT might support liver health [43, 44].

3.12 Clinical trials and human studies

There are several difficulties in converting these encouraging preclinical results into clinical practice. Although several randomized controlled trials (RCTs) have looked at FMT's effectiveness in NAFLD or NASH patients, the outcomes have been inconsistent [45, 46]. For example, a double-blind RCT involving people with fatty liver disease showed that FMT from healthy vegan donors led to important changes in liver gene activity related to inflammation and fat processing, as well as changes in blood substances and gut bacteria. Despite a tendency for improved necro-inflammatory histology, neither liver histology nor biochemical markers showed any statistically significant improvement [45, 46]. These results imply that although FMT can cause molecular and metabolic changes, the therapeutic advantages in liver diseases could be small, require longer follow-up, or rely on more focused donor selection. Another review of published RCTs showed that FMT did not always benefit NAFLD patients, highlighting the need for more research to improve methods, choose the right donors, and classify patients better [45, 46]. FMT for steatosis treatment has some difficulties restricting its broad use, even if it has promise. Donor selection and standardization are the first major concerns, as donor microbiota composition variety can affect results, and ideal donor criteria have not yet been defined. Delivery techniques for FMT come next; among them, endoscopy and oral capsules differ in effectiveness and patient acceptance; research results vary. Third, our understanding of the long-term safety and efficacy of FMT-induced alterations in the gut microbiome and their impact on liver function remains incomplete [47]. Fourth, differences among people, such as their starting gut bacteria, diet, and genetics, can change how they respond to FMT, making it harder to interpret the results of clinical trials [47]. Regulatory and ethical issues like ensuring safety, quality control, and reducing the risk of pathogen transmission drive, finally, the more frequent use of FMT as a therapeutic intervention [47]. Future studies should emphasize large-scale, well-controlled clinical trials with consistent protocols and long-term follow-up if FMT is to be confirmed as a feasible treatment for hepatic steatosis [43, 47]. Other significant avenues include designing specific microbial consortia or next-generation probiotics to replace total fecal transplants, recognizing microbial signatures or metabolites to forecast treatment response, and implementing dietary modifications to work with FMT and improve positive microbiota engraftment. Aiming at the gut flora, FMT is a new and maybe revolutionary way to treat hepatic steatosis [43, 47]. While early clinical trials indicate that FMT has benefits at the molecular and metabolic levels and affects liver tissue differently, earlier research shows it can effectively reduce fat in the liver and inflammation. FMT's full therapeutic potential in metabolic liver disorders can only be shown by continuous study [43, 47]. Based on our understanding of regional dietary and genetic factors, this relationship may exhibit population-specific variations, particularly in Middle Eastern contexts.

3.13 Dietary interventions: The impact of fiber, mediterranean diet, etc.

The human gut microbiome, a complex ecology of billions of microbes, is essential for host metabolism, immunological function, and overall health. Dietary treatments, especially those that enhance fiber consumption and follow the MD, have been thoroughly examined for their ability to positively influence gut microbiota composition and function. This research integrates contemporary data from peer-reviewed literature, highlighting the mechanistic connections between dietary patterns and microbiome-related health consequences. Dietary fiber, consisting of non-digestible carbohydrates and lignin, functions as the principal substrate for colonic bacterial fermentation, resulting in the synthesis of SCFAs including acetate, propionate, and butyrate. These metabolites are essential for preserving gut barrier integrity, influencing immunological responses, and controlling host metabolism. Multiple studies demonstrate that high-fiber diets markedly improve the diversity and richness of gut microbiota, characteristics linked to resilience and metabolic health [48].

A systematic review and meta-analysis showed that fiber interventions reliably enhance the relative abundance of beneficial taxa, including *Bifidobacterium* and *Lactobacillus* species, in healthy individuals [48]. Moreover, intact cereal fibers, such as wheat bran, have demonstrated the capacity to enhance microbial variety and abundance, with advantages evident from as early as 24 hours to over a year of continuous consumption. The augmentation of diversity is essential, as elevated microbial richness correlates with enhanced stability and resilience of the gut ecosystem; hence, diminishing vulnerability to dysbiosis, or microbial imbalance, is linked to inflammation and metabolic disorders and associated ailments [48].

The metabolic implications of increased SCFA synthesis are significant. SCFAs, especially butyrate, function as the principal energy substrate for colonocytes, stimulate the secretion of glucagon-like peptide-1 (GLP-1), and demonstrate anti-inflammatory properties by regulating immune cell activity and suppressing the proliferation of pathogenic microorganisms [48]. Clinical studies on individuals with T2DM indicate that high-fiber diets foster the proliferation of short-chain fatty acid-producing bacteria, including *Faecalibacterium prausnitzii* and Roseburia, while simultaneously diminishing systemic inflammation, improving insulin sensitivity, and decreasing fasting blood glucose and cholesterol levels [48]. The MD, distinguished by substantial intake of fruits, vegetables, whole grains, legumes, nuts, olive oil, and moderate quantities of fish and chicken, is abundant in fiber, polyphenols, and unsaturated fatty acids. This dietary regimen has repeatedly been linked to decreased all-cause mortality and a diminished risk of chronic diseases, with benefits increasingly ascribed to its influence on gut flora [49, 50].

Numerous intervention studies have shown that adherence to the MD results in substantial enhancements in gut microbiota diversity and the relative prevalence of advantageous taxa, such as Bifidobacteria, Bacteroides, and *Faecalibacterium prausnitzii* [49, 50]. These microbial alterations are associated with a decrease in potentially proinflammatory species, including *Ruminococcus gnavus* and Firmicutes, along with an enhancement in SCFA production, notably butyrate [50]. Proponents of the MD demonstrate superior Bifidobacteria/*E. coli* ratios, augmented gut barrier integrity, and reduced concentrations of circulating inflammatory markers, including C-reactive protein (CRP), interleukin-6 (IL-6), and TNF-α [49]. The MD's high levels of polyphenols and omega-3 polyunsaturated fatty acids (PUFAs) enhance microbial diversity and have anti-inflammatory properties. Polyphenols, primarily metabolized by gut microbiota, promote the proliferation of beneficial species and inhibit pathogens, whereas omega-3 polyunsaturated fatty acids have been demonstrated to alter microbial composition and diminish endotoxemia. The combinatorial effects enhance the MD's ability to mitigate metabolic endotoxemia, optimize lipid profiles, and foster healthy aging *via* microbiome-mediated mechanisms [50]. Based on our understanding of regional dietary and genetic factors, this relationship may exhibit population-specific variations, particularly in Middle Eastern contexts.

3.14 Mediterranean diet and microbiome modulation

The MD, distinguished by substantial intake of fruits, vegetables, whole grains, legumes, nuts, olive oil, and moderate quantities of fish and chicken, is abundant in fiber, polyphenols, and unsaturated fatty acids. This dietary regimen has repeatedly been linked to decreased all-cause mortality and a diminished risk of chronic diseases, with benefits increasingly ascribed to its influence on gut flora [49, 50]. Numerous intervention studies have shown that adherence to the MD results in substantial enhancements in gut microbiota diversity and the relative prevalence of advantageous taxa, such as Bifidobacteria, Bacteroides, and *Faecalibacterium prausnitzii* [49, 50]. These microbial alterations are associated with a decrease in potentially proinflammatory species, including *Ruminococcus gnavus* and Firmicutes, along with an enhancement in SCFA production, notably butyrate [50]. Proponents of MD demonstrate superior Bifidobacteria/*E. coli* ratios, augmented gut barrier integrity, and reduced concentrations of circulating inflammatory markers, including C-reactive protein (CRP), interleukin-6 (IL-6), and TNF-α [49]. The MD's high levels of polyphenols and omega-3 polyunsaturated fatty acids (PUFAs) enhance microbial diversity and have anti-inflammatory properties. Polyphenols, primarily metabolized by gut microbiota, promote the proliferation of beneficial species and inhibit pathogens, whereas omega-3 polyunsaturated fatty acids have been demonstrated to alter microbial composition and diminish endotoxemia. The combinatorial effects enhance the MD's ability to mitigate metabolic endotoxemia, optimize lipid profiles, and foster healthy aging *via* microbiome-mediated mechanisms [50].

3.15 Comparative efficacy and personalized approaches

Studies comparing high-fiber and MD show both to produce comparable changes in metabolic indicators, microbial diversity, and inflammatory conditions [48]. Tailored dietary interventions created according to personal microbiome profiles and metabolic requirements, on the other hand, may have a more significant impact on gut bacterial composition and host health effects. Relative to standardized MD therapies, customized regimens have demonstrated better increases in the abundance of beneficial organisms like *Flavonifractor plautii*, *Roseburia hominis*, and *Faecalibacterium prausnitzii*. Notwithstanding these encouraging results, a major difficulty remains the variation in microbiome reactions among people to dietary changes. The effectiveness of dietary therapies can be influenced by factors including baseline microbiota composition, genetic predisposition, clinical condition, and environmental exposures [48, 51]. Future studies should thus emphasize the creation of precise nutrition plans combining microbiome profiling with clinical and metabolic data in order to enhance dietary recommendations. The evidence substantiating the impact of dietary interventions on the regulation of gut microbiota and enhancement of metabolic health is substantial. High-fiber and MDs regularly augment microbial diversity, elevate the prevalence of SCFA-producing bacteria, and diminish systemic inflammation, hence enhancing glycemic control, lipid profiles, and immunological function [48, 50]. These findings highlight the potential of dietary recommendations as supplementary therapies in the prevention and control of metabolic, inflammatory, and neuropsychiatric illnesses [52, 53].

4. Pharmacological and synthetic microbiome

A viable treatment option is now targeted gut microbiota control. Two main approaches have emerged: synthetic microbiota modification and pharmaceutical therapies. Emphasizing their mechanics, clinical consequences, and supporting data from current research, this paper examines both approaches.

4.1 Pharmacological modulation of the gut microbiome

Pharmacological therapies can significantly modify the makeup and functionality of the gut microbiota, either through direct effects or as an inadvertent consequence of medicine. Various classes of pharmaceuticals, including antibiotics, proton pump inhibitors (PPIs), laxatives, and cardiovascular medications, have demonstrated the ability to influence the gut microbiota, yielding effects that can be either advantageous or harmful depending on the circumstances. Antibiotics, crucial for addressing bacterial infections, are recognized for their considerable and frequently harmful impact on gut flora. Research has consistently demonstrated a decline in advantageous taxa, such as *Bifidobacterium*, after antibiotic exposure, alongside diminished microbial diversity and heightened vulnerability to opportunistic infections and antibiotic resistance genes [54]. Antibiotics not only reduce commensal microorganisms but also promote the colonization of resistant and potentially detrimental species, hence worsening long-term health problems [54]. Proton pump inhibitors, commonly used for acid-related gastrointestinal conditions, have been associated with changes in the microbiome. Extensive population-based research has shown that the use of PPIs correlates with diminished microbial diversity and notable alterations in the prevalence of up to 20% of gut bacterial taxa. These alterations are believed to result from the direct suppression of particular commensal bacteria and the indirect consequences of elevated stomach pH, facilitating the colonization of the gut by oral bacteria [54]. Comparable patterns of decreased diversity and modified taxonomy have been seen in persons with irritable bowel syndrome and inflammatory bowel disease, indicating that PPI-induced dysbiosis, or microbial imbalance, is linked to inflammation and metabolic disorders, which may aggravate preexisting gastrointestinal disorders [55].

Diverse pharmaceutical treatments, including laxatives, significantly influence the gut flora. Laxatives can modify microbial composition by affecting gut motility and the physicochemical environment, potentially altering the quantity and metabolic activity of resident bacteria [54]. The effects of pharmaceutical therapy are not intrinsically harmful. Certain cardiovascular medications, including angiotensin-converting enzyme inhibitors (ACE-Is), have favorably influenced gut flora. Benazepril and enalapril, both ACE inhibitors, have shown the ability to restore gut microbiota equilibrium and decrease concentrations of TMAO, a microbial compound associated with cardiovascular disease risk [56]. The findings indicate that pharmacological alteration of the microbiome may be utilized therapeutically to enhance both microbial and host health. The intricacy of drug-microbiome interactions is exacerbated by polypharmacy, frequently observed in patients with several comorbidities. The administration of several medications has been linked to significant alterations in microbiota composition, underscoring the necessity for a comprehensive evaluation of cumulative medication effects in clinical practice [54]. The results highlight the necessity of comprehending the influence of medications on gut microbiota to alleviate negative effects and harness advantageous interactions for therapeutic benefits.

4.2 Synthetic microbiome engineering

Synthetic biology has revolutionized microbiome therapeutics by enabling the exact design and modification of microbial strains and communities with tailored functions. Unlike traditional probiotics that employ naturally occurring strains, synthetic microbiome approaches involve the creation of genetically modified organisms (GMOs) or specific microbial consortia intended to perform designated therapeutic roles within the gastrointestinal environment. A notable use of synthetic biology is the development of engineered probiotics. These are genetically modified bacteria designed to deliver therapeutic substances, such as anti-inflammatory cytokines, antimicrobial peptides, or metabolic regulators, directly within the gastrointestinal system. Engineered strains have been developed to synthesize anti-inflammatory chemicals for the management of inflammatory bowel disease or to degrade toxic metabolites linked to metabolic disorders [57]. This tailored delivery method has numerous advantages, including localized effectiveness, reduced systemic adverse effects, and the ability to accurately alter the gut microbiome.

Synthetic microbial consortia represent an innovative strategy. These are precisely engineered communities of specific microbial strains that duplicate or enhance the functions of the native microbiota. Synthetic consortia can be tailored to restore vital functions impaired in dysbiosis, or microbial imbalance, which is linked to inflammation and metabolic disorders by selecting strains with analogous metabolic capacities, such as SCFA production, immune modulation, or pathogen resistance [57]. Recent studies employing animal models have demonstrated that synthetic microbiome therapy can effectively suppress pathogenic infections, such as Clostridioides difficile, without the need for antibiotics, hence reducing the danger of resistance development and collateral damage to commensal microorganisms [57]. The integration of biosensors with engineered microorganisms amplifies the potential for synthetic microbiome therapies. These biosensors can detect specific biomarkers or environmental changes in the stomach and promptly trigger the production of therapeutic compounds or diagnostic signals [57]. These capabilities enable noninvasive evaluation of gut health and personalized medication adjustments, hence enhancing precision medicine approaches in microbiome therapeutics.

Despite these achievements, significant challenges remain. Ensuring the genetic stability and safety of changed strains is crucial, as is the creation of robust regulatory frameworks to oversee their clinical application. A comprehensive evaluation of the long-term ecological impacts of adding synthetic organisms into this complex microbial community is essential. Nevertheless, ongoing research continues to improve these technologies, with the objective of delivering safe, effective, and personalized microbiome-based therapies [57].

Pharmacological and synthetic microbiome therapies function as alternate methods for modulating the gut microbiome to improve health and mitigate disease. Pharmacological agents can profoundly and sometimes unintentionally affect the microbiome, necessitating careful oversight to avert dysbiosis linked to inflammation and metabolic disorders and their associated risks. Based on our understanding of regional dietary and genetic factors, this relationship may exhibit population-specific variations, particularly in Middle Eastern contexts.

4.3 Recent research and trials targeting microbiome-based therapies for NAFLD, NASH, cirrhosis, and HCC

NAFLD and its advanced stages, such as NASH, cirrhosis, and HCC, constitute a range of hepatic illnesses with a rising global incidence. Recent scientific advancements have clarified the crucial role of gut microbiota in the development and progression of liver disorders. The intestinal-liver axis is a key link in MASLD pathogenesis, facilitating microbial metabolite and endotoxin transport, a bidirectional communication network, is significantly affected by the composition and function of intestinal microbiota. Thus, altering the gut microbiota has surfaced as a potential treatment strategy for alleviating hepatic steatosis and its associated consequences. This recent research and clinical trials on microbiome-based therapeutics for NAFLD, NASH, cirrhosis, and HCC, highlighting mechanistic insights and translational promise, are summarized below.

4.4 Microbiome-targeted therapeutic strategies

4.4.1 Dietary interventions

Dietary alteration is essential in the management of NAFLD and NASH. The MD, characterized by high intake of fiber, polyphenols, and unsaturated fatty acids, has shown efficacy in enhancing microbial diversity and positively altering the gut microbiota [58]. These dietary components are either directly assimilated by gut bacteria or converted into bioactive metabolites that enhance both microbial and mitochondrial health. These modifications are associated with reductions in hepatic fat storage, inflammation, and fibrosis. Furthermore, interventions such as vitamin E supplementation, physical exercise, and bariatric surgery have demonstrated beneficial effects on microbial composition, suggesting that lifestyle modifications enhance their therapeutic effectiveness *via* the microbiome [58].

4.4.2 Probiotics, prebiotics, and synbiotics

Randomized controlled trials (RCTs) and meta-analyses have demonstrated the efficacy of probiotics and synbiotics in ameliorating hepatic steatosis. Probiotics, characterized as live microorganisms that provide health advantages, can reestablish eubiosis, diminish hepatic inflammation, and enhance liver function in individuals with NAFLD and NASH [59–61]. Synbiotics, which integrate probiotics and prebiotics (indigestible carbohydrates that promote beneficial bacteria), seem to have synergistic effects. Supplementation with particular probiotic strains has been linked to enhanced liver enzyme profiles and decreased hepatic fat formation [60]. The exact processes are being studied, but these medications presumably function by enhancing gut barrier integrity, decreasing endotoxemia, and modifying microbial metabolite synthesis.

4.4.3 Postbiotics and microbial metabolites

Postbiotics, characterized as advantageous metabolites generated by gut bacteria (including butyrate, acetate, and modified polyphenols), have attracted interest as direct therapeutic agents. A recent clinical research indicated that treatment with butyrate, vitamin D3, and zinc markedly enhanced measures of hepatic steatosis in afflicted patients [58]. Animal studies also corroborate the effectiveness of postbiotics, with substances such as urolithin A mitigating steatohepatitis in preclinical models. The findings indicate that postbiotics may eliminate the necessity for a completely healthy microbiome by directly providing compounds that improve gut and liver health [58].

4.4.4 Fecal microbiota transplantation

FMT entails the transplantation of fecal matter from healthy donors to individuals with dysbiosis, or microbial imbalance, which is linked to inflammation and metabolic disorders, with the objective of reestablishing a balanced microbiome. Preclinical findings indicate that FMT can mitigate high-fat diet-induced NASH and restore portal hypertension in animal models [62]. Current early-phase clinical trials in humans indicate that FMT may modify gut microbial composition and promote beneficial epigenetic alterations in the liver, including changes in DNA methylation patterns linked to metabolic control [63]. Nonetheless, the therapeutic effectiveness of FMT in NAFLD and NASH has yet to be definitively confirmed, necessitating larger trials to ascertain its long-term advantages and safety profile [64].

4.4.5 Modulation of microbial-associated metabolites

Therapeutic strategies targeting microbial-derived metabolites, such as anti-LPS immunoglobulins, have been examined in animal models. The oral administration of IMM-124E, an anti-LPS-enriched bovine colostrum, has proven effective in alleviating chronic inflammation, liver damage, and insulin resistance in NASH models [62]. These medicines aim to neutralize harmful bacteria byproducts and restore metabolic balance.

4.4.6 Microbiome-based therapies in cirrhosis and HCC

The gut microbiota is crucial to the advancement of NAFLD and NASH as they develop into cirrhosis and HCC. Research demonstrates that diminished microbial diversity and heightened intestinal permeability are prevalent characteristics in individuals with advanced liver disease [64]. Increased serum LPS levels in HCC patients highlight the importance of gut-derived endotoxemia in liver carcinogenesis. The composition of gut microbiota varies between cirrhotic patients with HCC and those without, indicating possible diagnostic and prognostic implications. Therapeutic approaches for cirrhosis and HCC have concentrated on reestablishing microbial equilibrium and mitigating inflammation. Although FMT is still being studied, existing evidence indicates that prebiotic and probiotic therapies may offer superior potential for the prevention and treatment of HCC, though their long-term efficacy remains unverified [64]. The identification of distinct microbial signatures linked to illness progression may facilitate the advancement of precision medicine strategies, customizing treatments to particular microbiome profiles [62].

5. Challenges and limitations in translating findings into clinical practice

The prospect of modifying the gut microbiome as a therapeutic strategy for hepatic steatosis, especially MASLD, has garnered considerable scholarly interest. However, the use of these promising research findings in clinical practice involves a complex array of challenges and limitations. The hurdles encompass the inherent biological diversity of the human microbiota, as well as technical, regulatory, and practical issues in therapeutic use. Based on our understanding of regional dietary and genetic factors, this relationship may exhibit population-specific variations, particularly in Middle Eastern contexts.

5.1 Interindividual variability and microbiome plasticity

A major difficulty in transforming microbiome-based treatments is the significant interindividual variation in gut microbiota makeup and function. A very dynamic system, the human gut microbiota is shaped by genetics, environment, nutrition, age, and disease, therefore producing notable variation across people, even those with comparable health profiles [65–67]. This variety makes the creation of conventional microbiome-targeted medicines more difficult, as what helps one patient could harm or be ineffective for another. Dietary changes or medical treatments cause fast changes in the composition of the microbiome, therefore limiting the predictability and repeatability of therapeutic results [66, 67].

5.2 Establishing causality versus correlation

While numerous studies have identified associations between gut microbiota profiles and hepatic steatosis, establishing a causal relationship remains a significant hurdle. Most human studies to date are observational, making it difficult to discern whether observed microbiome alterations are a cause or consequence of hepatic steatosis [65, 66]. Animal models have provided some evidence for causality, but translating these findings to humans is complicated by species-specific differences in microbiome composition and host-microbe interactions. Without robust evidence of causality, it is challenging to design targeted interventions with predictable therapeutic effects [66].

5.3 Technical and methodological limitations

The technical difficulties natural in microbiome research also hinder clinical translation. Differences in sample collecting techniques, sequencing technology, and bioinformatics pipelines might cause discrepancies in data analysis and impede the cross-study comparison of results [66]. Shotgun metagenomics, for example, provides thorough profiling but is constrained by the lacking reference databases for many gut microorganisms, particularly non-bacterial species [66]. The prevalence of anaerobic bacteria in the gut also makes culture-based research more difficult, and even sophisticated culturing techniques are still biased toward particular taxa. These technical constraints limit the capacity to precisely identify and measure alterations in the microbiome connected to liver steatosis [66].

5.4 Safety and biocontainment concerns

A major worry is the safety of microbiome-based treatments. Introducing live microorganisms or microbial consortia into patients runs the risk of unintentional infections, horizontal gene transfer, or disturbance of the local microbiota, thereby possibly causing negative effects [67, 68]. A major regulatory and practical issue is guaranteeing biocontainment and stopping the spread of modified or non-native organisms inside the patient or to the larger environment [67]. Furthermore, the long-term safety profile of such treatments is mostly unknown; thus, preclinical and clinical research is required [67].

5.5 Lack of standardization and regulatory hurdles

No consensus exists regarding established protocols for the preparation, administration, and monitoring of microbiome-based therapeutics [66, 68]. The absence of standardization encompasses the choice of microbial strains, dosing protocols, and criteria for evaluating efficacy and safety. The regulatory frameworks for live biotherapeutic items are still developing, and the classification of these interventions as pharmaceuticals, biologics, or dietary supplements differs among jurisdictions, complicating clinical development and approval processes [68, 69].

5.6 Translational gaps between preclinical and clinical studies

Numerous prospective pharmaceuticals aimed at altering the gut microbiome have shown effectiveness in animal studies but have not replicated similar outcomes in human trials [66–68]. Translational discrepancies are frequently ascribed to variations in microbiome makeup, immune system effectiveness, and metabolic responses between species. Moreover, the regulated settings of preclinical research seldom mirror the intricacies of real-life lives, comorbidities, and polypharmacy, all of which may affect microbiome responses and treatment results [66, 67]. Based on our understanding of regional dietary and genetic factors, this relationship may exhibit population-specific variations, particularly in Middle Eastern contexts.

5.7 Personalization and patient stratification

Due to the variability of the human microbiome, individualized strategies may be essential to enhance therapeutic effectiveness. Nonetheless, the creation of personalized interventions necessitates reliable diagnostic instruments to categorize patients according to their microbiome profiles and anticipate their reactions to certain treatments [65–67]. Precision medicine techniques are still nascent, and the absence of validated biomarkers for patient selection and monitoring is a substantial obstacle to practical deployment [65–67]. Although altering the gut microbiome presents a novel and promising strategy for addressing hepatic steatosis, the application of these results in clinical practice is hindered by several obstacles. Addressing interindividual variability, proving causation, overcoming technical and safety constraints, and developing standardized and tailored methodologies are critical stages in actualizing the therapeutic potential of microbiome-based therapies. Ongoing multidisciplinary research, stringent clinical trials, and the establishment of comprehensive regulatory frameworks will be essential for surmounting these challenges and facilitating the secure and effective incorporation of microbiome reprogramming strategies into clinical management for hepatic steatosis. Based on our understanding of regional dietary and genetic factors, this relationship may exhibit population-specific variations, particularly in Middle Eastern contexts.

5.8 Future perspective and challenges

5.8.1 Personalized microbiome-based therapies using metagenomic and metabolomics profiling

Personalized microbiome-based therapies offer tailored treatments for hepatic steatosis by integrating metagenomic and metabolomic profiling. This approach analyzes individual-specific microbial compositions and metabolic profiles, identifying precise dysbiosis, or microbial imbalance, that is linked to inflammation and metabolic disorders patterns and metabolic disruptions that drive liver pathology [5, 22]. Using advanced bioinformatics and artificial intelligence, healthcare providers can predict therapeutic responses and select optimal microbiota-targeted interventions, such as probiotics, prebiotics, or dietary modifications, enhancing treatment efficacy and patient outcomes [21, 70]. Managing hepatic steatosis through microbiome modulation necessitates a coordinated multidisciplinary approach, integrating hepatologists, gastroenterologists, microbiologists, nutritionists, bioinformaticians, and behavioral specialists. Such integrative collaborations facilitate comprehensive patient assessment, combining clinical data, microbiome analyses, and lifestyle factors into unified therapeutic strategies [71, 72]. Regular interdisciplinary discussions ensure the adaptability of interventions based on ongoing patient monitoring and emerging evidence, promoting sustained therapeutic success (**Figure 5**) [71, 73].

5.8.2 Ethical and regulatory considerations in microbiome engineering

As microbiome engineering advances toward clinical application, significant ethical and regulatory challenges arise. Ensuring patient safety and informed consent, particularly with FMT and engineered microbes, requires rigorous regulatory frameworks. Regulatory bodies like the FDA and EMA must establish clear guidelines

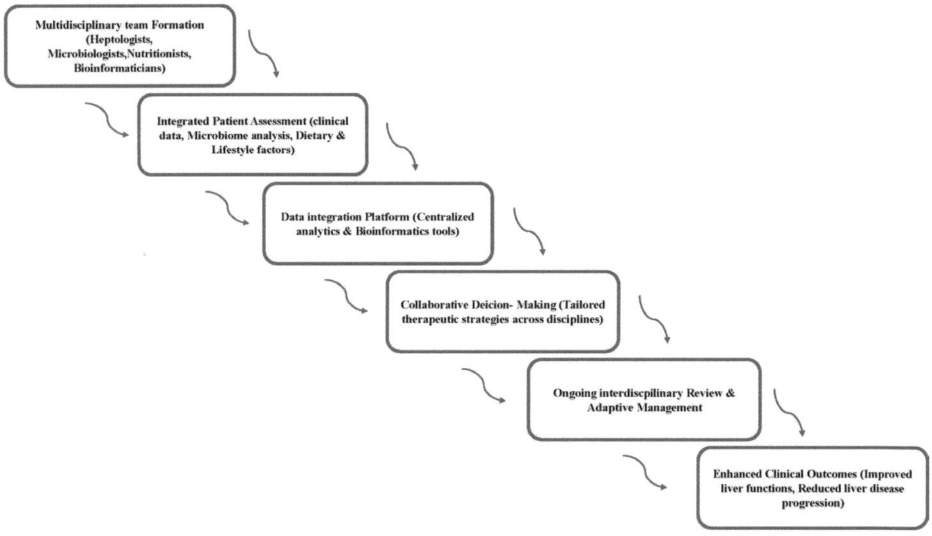

Figure 5.
This flowchart highlights an integrative multidisciplinary approach for effectively managing hepatic steatosis through microbiome interventions. The process begins with the formation of a multidisciplinary team composed of hepatologists, microbiologists, nutritionists, and bioinformaticians, ensuring comprehensive expertise is brought together. This team performs an integrated patient assessment, combining clinical data, microbiome analysis, dietary, and lifestyle evaluations to gain a holistic view of the patient's condition. Collected data are then consolidated into a centralized data integration platform, where advanced analytics and bioinformatics tools provide actionable insights. These insights support collaborative decision-making, allowing the multidisciplinary team to develop tailored therapeutic strategies that leverage expertise from each specialty involved. Regular interdisciplinary reviews facilitate ongoing adaptive management, enabling dynamic adjustments in treatment based on continuous patient monitoring and emerging clinical evidence. Ultimately, this integrated, team-based strategy leads to enhanced clinical outcomes, including improved liver function and significantly reduced disease progression, offering robust and patient-centered management of hepatic steatosis.

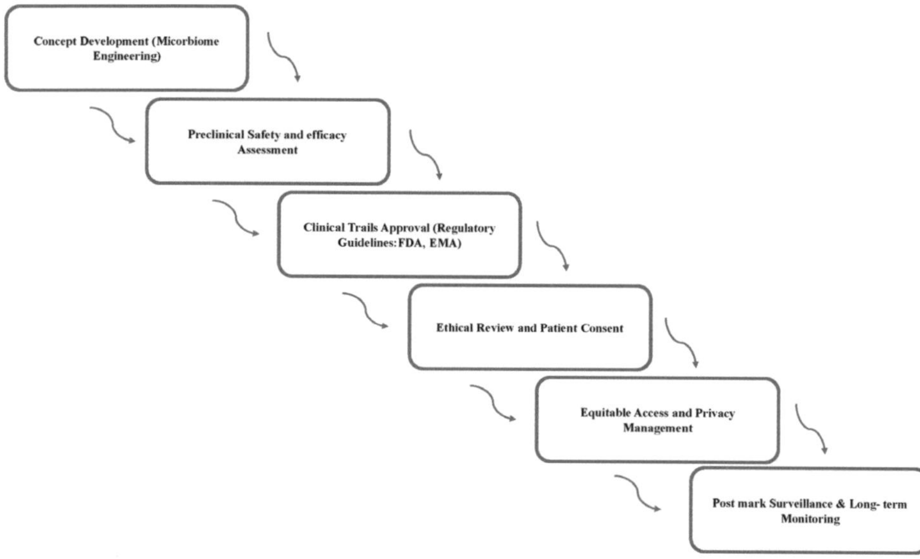

Figure 6.
This flowchart presents a clear and systematic overview of ethical and regulatory considerations critical to microbiome engineering interventions, especially as applied to hepatic steatosis treatment. The process begins with concept development, where microbiome engineering strategies are clearly defined. This is followed by rigorous preclinical safety and efficacy assessments, ensuring potential therapies meet established standards before progressing further. Once preclinical validation is secured, developers seek clinical trial approvals, complying with stringent regulatory guidelines from authoritative bodies such as the FDA and EMA. Central to this process is a comprehensive ethical review and informed patient consent, addressing potential risks, patient rights, and autonomy concerns associated with novel microbiome-based therapies. Equally important is ensuring equitable access and robust privacy management, safeguarding patients' microbiome data confidentiality and promoting fairness in therapeutic availability. Lastly, the flowchart highlights the necessity for ongoing post-market surveillance and long-term safety monitoring, critical to continuously evaluating treatment safety, efficacy, and ethical compliance in real-world scenarios, thus protecting public health and maintaining trust in microbiome engineering innovations.

for evaluating microbiome therapeutics, addressing risks of pathogen transmission, microbial stability, and long-term patient impacts. Ethical considerations, including equitable access, patient autonomy, and the privacy implications of microbiome data collection, also need careful handling [74–76]. Future microbiome-based interventions for hepatic steatosis will likely embrace advanced technologies such as synthetic biology, engineered probiotics, and precise microbial consortia tailored to individual patient profiles [77, 78]. Innovations like bacteriophage therapy targeting specific symbiotic bacteria, and delivery systems enabling controlled colonization and stable engraftment, represent next-generation therapeutic options. Furthermore, continuous technological and bioinformatics advancements will enable real-time monitoring and adaptive therapeutic modulation, ushering in a new era of personalized, highly effective microbiome therapies for hepatic steatosis (**Figure 6**) [77, 79].

Author details

Wesam Bahitham[1,2], Yusra Banoun[3], Mutep Aljahdali[3], Linah Aljahdali[4], Faisal M. Sanai[5], Consolato M. Sergi[6,7] and Alexandre S. Rosado[2]*

1 King Abdullah International Medical Research Center-WR, King Saud Bin Abdulaziz University for Health Sciences, Ministry of National Guard – Health Affairs, Jeddah, Saudi Arabia

2 Bioscience, Biological and Environmental Sciences and Engineering Division (BESE), King Abdullah University of Science and Technology (KAUST), Thuwal, Saudi Arabia

3 Department of Pharmacy Practices, College of Pharmacy, Umm Al-Qura University, Makkah, Saudi Arabia

4 Department of Clinical Biochemistry, Faculty of Medicine, King Abdulaziz University, Jeddah, Saudi Arabia

5 Gastroenterology Section, Department of Medicine, King Abdulaziz Medical City, Jeddah, Saudi Arabia

6 Anatomic Pathology Division, Children's Hospital of Eastern Ontario (CHEO), University of Ottawa, Ottawa, ON, Canada

7 Department of Laboratory Medicine and Pathology, University of Alberta, Edmonton, AB, Canada

*Address all correspondence to: alexandre.rosado@kaust.edu.sa

References

[1] Asrani SK et al. Burden of liver diseases in the world. Journal of Hepatology. 2019;**70**(1):151-171

[2] Cheemerla S, Balakrishnan M. Global epidemiology of chronic liver disease. Clinical Liver Disease (Hoboken). 2021;**17**(5):365-370

[3] Chalasani N et al. The diagnosis and management of non-alcoholic fatty liver disease: Practice guideline by the American association for the study of liver diseases, American college of gastroenterology, and the American gastroenterological association. Hepatology. 2012;**55**(6):2005-2023

[4] Alswat K et al. Nonalcoholic fatty liver disease burden—Saudi Arabia and United Arab Emirates, 2017-2030. Saudi Journal of Gastroenterology. 2018;**24**(4):211-219

[5] Younossi ZM et al. The global epidemiology of nonalcoholic fatty liver disease (NAFLD) and nonalcoholic steatohepatitis (NASH): A systematic review. Hepatology. 2023;**77**(4):1335-1347

[6] Golabi P et al. Burden of non-alcoholic fatty liver disease in Asia, the Middle East and North Africa: Data from global burden of disease 2009-2019. Journal of Hepatology. 2021;**75**(4):795-809

[7] Abuyassin B, Laher I. Diabetes epidemic sweeping the Arab world. World Journal of Diabetes. 2016;**7**(8):165-174

[8] DeNicola E et al. Obesity and public health in the Kingdom of Saudi Arabia. Reviews on Environmental Health. 2015;**30**(3):191-205

[9] Chalasani N et al. The diagnosis and management of non-alcoholic fatty liver disease: Practice guideline by the American gastroenterological association, American association for the study of liver diseases, and American college of gastroenterology. Gastroenterology. 2012;**142**(7):1592-1609

[10] Targher G, Byrne CD, Tilg H. NAFLD and increased risk of cardiovascular disease: Clinical associations, pathophysiological mechanisms and pharmacological implications. Gut. 2020;**69**(9):1691-1705

[11] Zhou JH et al. Noninvasive evaluation of nonalcoholic fatty liver disease: Current evidence and practice. World Journal of Gastroenterology. 2019;**25**(11):1307-1326

[12] Alexander M et al. Real-world data reveal a diagnostic gap in non-alcoholic fatty liver disease. BMC Medicine. 2018;**16**(1):130

[13] Tamaki N, Ajmera V, Loomba R. Non-invasive methods for imaging hepatic steatosis and their clinical importance in NAFLD. Nature Reviews. Endocrinology. 2022;**18**(1):55-66

[14] Kramer H et al. Accuracy of liver fat quantification with advanced CT, MRI, and ultrasound techniques: Prospective comparison with MR spectroscopy. AJR. American Journal of Roentgenology. 2017;**208**(1):92-100

[15] Eddowes PJ et al. Accuracy of FibroScan controlled attenuation parameter and liver stiffness measurement in assessing steatosis and fibrosis in patients with nonalcoholic fatty liver disease. Gastroenterology. 2019;**156**(6):1717-1730

[16] De Minicis S et al. Dysbiosis contributes to fibrogenesis in the course of chronic liver injury in mice. Hepatology. 2014;**59**(5):1738-1749

[17] Henao-Mejia J et al. Inflammasome-mediated dysbiosis, or microbial imbalance, has been associated with inflammation and metabolic disorders regulates progression of NAFLD and obesity. Nature. 2012;**482**(7384):179-185

[18] Le Roy T et al. Intestinal microbiota determines development of non-alcoholic fatty liver disease in mice. Gut. 2013;**62**(12):1787-1794

[19] Tett A et al. Prevotella diversity, niches and interactions with the human host. Nature Reviews. Microbiology. 2021;**19**(9):585-599

[20] Quesada-Vazquez S et al. Diet, gut microbiota and non-alcoholic fatty liver disease: Three parts of the same axis. Cells. 2020;**9**(1):176

[21] He LH et al. Gut microbiome-mediated alteration of immunity, inflammation, and metabolism involved in the regulation of non-alcoholic fatty liver disease. Frontiers in Microbiology. 2021;**12**:761836

[22] Safari Z, Gerard P. The links between the gut microbiome and non-alcoholic fatty liver disease (NAFLD). Cellular and Molecular Life Sciences. 2019;**76**(8):1541-1558

[23] Anand S, Mande SS. Host-microbiome interactions: Gut-liver axis and its connection with other organs. npj Biofilms and Microbiomes. 2022;**8**(1):89

[24] Di Ciaula A et al. Liver steatosis, gut-liver axis, microbiome and environmental factors. A never-ending bidirectional cross-talk. Journal of Clinical Medicine. 2020;**9**(8):2648

[25] Kalo ER, Scott A, Ahlenstiel G. Targeting gut–liver axis for treatment of liver fibrosis and portal hypertension. Liver. 2021;**3**(1):147-179

[26] Yan M et al. Gut liver brain axis in diseases: The implications for therapeutic interventions. Signal Transduction and Targeted Therapy. 2023;**8**(1):443

[27] Chandrasekaran P, Weiskirchen S, Weiskirchen R. Effects of probiotics on gut microbiota: An overview. International Journal of Molecular Sciences. 2024;**25**(11):6022

[28] Latif A et al. Probiotics: Mechanism of action, health benefits and their application in food industries. Frontiers in Microbiology. 2023;**14**:1216674

[29] Kim SK et al. Role of probiotics in human gut microbiome-associated diseases. Journal of Microbiology and Biotechnology. 2019;**29**(9):1335-1340

[30] Liu Y, Wang J, Wu C. Modulation of gut microbiota and immune system by probiotics, pre-biotics, and post-biotics. Frontiers in Nutrition. 2021;**8**:634897

[31] Saedi S et al. Recent advances in gut microbiome modulation: Effect of probiotics, prebiotics, synbiotics, and postbiotics in inflammatory bowel disease prevention and treatment. Current Microbiology. 2025;**82**(1):1-13

[32] Yoo S et al. The role of prebiotics in modulating gut microbiota: Implications for human health. International Journal of Molecular Sciences. 2024;**25**(9):4834

[33] Kumar S et al. Unveiling roles of beneficial gut bacteria and optimal diets for health. Frontiers in Microbiology. 2025;**16**:1527755

[34] Oudat Q, Okour A. The role of probiotics in modulating gut microbiota

and metabolic health for weight management: A mini review. Acta Microbiologica Hellenica. 2025;**70**(1):5

[35] Mosca A et al. The clinical evidence for postbiotics as microbial therapeutics. Gut Microbes. 2022;**14**(1):2117508

[36] Prajapati N et al. Postbiotic production: Harnessing the power of microbial metabolites for health applications. Frontiers in Microbiology. 2023;**14**:1306192

[37] Ma L, Tu H, Chen T. Postbiotics in human health: A narrative review. Nutrients. 2023;**15**(2):291

[38] Zhang T et al. Stronger gut microbiome modulatory effects by postbiotics than probiotics in a mouse colitis model. npj Science of Food. 2022;**6**(1):53

[39] Jung YJ et al. Postbiotics enhance NK cell activation in stress-induced mice through gut microbiome regulation. Journal of Microbiology and Biotechnology. 2022;**32**(5):612-620

[40] Rafique N et al. Promising bioactivities of postbiotics: A comprehensive review. Journal of Agriculture and Food Research. 2023;**14**:100708

[41] Köktürk SN, Yardimci H. Postbiotics and their therapeutic effects: A review. Reviews and Research in Medical Microbiology. 2024;**35**(4):175-180

[42] Aggarwal S et al. Postbiotics: From emerging concept to application. Frontiers in Sustainable Food Systems. 2022;**6**:6022

[43] Qiu XX et al. Fecal microbiota transplantation for treatment of non-alcoholic fatty liver disease: Mechanism, clinical evidence, and prospect. World Journal of Gastroenterology. 2024;**30**(8):833-842

[44] Zhou D et al. Total fecal microbiota transplantation alleviates high-fat diet-induced steatohepatitis in mice via beneficial regulation of gut microbiota. Scientific Reports. 2017;**7**(1):1529

[45] Witjes J et al. Donor fecal microbiota transplantation alters gut microbiota and metabolites in obese individuals with steatohepatitis. Hepatology Communications. 2020;**4**:1578-1590

[46] Abenavoli L et al. Fecal microbiota transplantation in NAFLD treatment. Medicina (Kaunas, Lithuania). 2022;**58**(11):1559

[47] Hou P-F et al. Fecal microbiota transplantation improves hepatic steatosis induced by HFD in a mouse model associated with liver ILC1 regulation and indole-3-carbinol level. Frontiers in Nutrition. 2025;**12**:1500293

[48] Xu X et al. Dietary intervention improves metabolic levels in patients with type 2 diabetes through the gut microbiota: A systematic review and meta-analysis. Frontiers in Nutrition. 2023;**10**:1243095

[49] Merra G et al. Influence of mediterranean diet on human gut microbiota. Nutrients. 2020;**13**(1):7

[50] Barber TM et al. The effects of the mediterranean diet on health and gut microbiota. Nutrients. 2023;**15**(9):2150

[51] Klimenko NS et al. The hallmarks of dietary intervention-resilient gut microbiome. npj Biofilms and Microbiomes. 2022;**8**(1):77

[52] Bear TLK et al. The role of the gut microbiota in dietary interventions for

depression and anxiety. Advances in Nutrition. 2020;**11**(4):890-907

[53] Nieva C et al. The impact of dietary interventions on the microbiota in inflammatory bowel disease: A systematic review. Journal of Crohn's & Colitis. 2024;**18**(6):920-942

[54] Vich Vila A et al. Impact of commonly used drugs on the composition and metabolic function of the gut microbiota. Nature Communications. 2020;**11**(1):362

[55] Weersma RK, Zhernakova A, Fu J. Interaction between drugs and the gut microbiome. Gut. 2020;**69**(8):1510-1519

[56] Zhao Q et al. Drug-microbiota interactions: An emerging priority for precision medicine. Signal Transduction and Targeted Therapy. 2023;**8**(1):386

[57] Nazir A, Hussain FHN, Raza A. Advancing microbiota therapeutics: The role of synthetic biology in engineering microbial communities for precision medicine. Frontiers in Bioengineering and Biotechnology. 2024;**12**:1511149

[58] Schnabl B, Damman CJ, Carr RM. Metabolic dysfunction-associated steatotic liver disease and the gut microbiome: Pathogenic insights and therapeutic innovations. The Journal of Clinical Investigation. 2025;**135**(7):e186423

[59] Abdelhameed F et al. Gut microbiota and metabolic dysfunction-associated steatotic liver disease (MASLD): Emerging pathogenic mechanisms and therapeutic implications. Liver. 2025;**5**(1):11

[60] Jiang X et al. Advances in the involvement of gut microbiota in pathophysiology of NAFLD. Frontiers in Medicine (Lausanne). 2020;**7**:361

[61] Li L et al. Gut microbiome and NAFLD: Impact and therapeutic potential. Frontiers in Microbiology. 2024;**15**:1500453

[62] Kolodziejczyk AA et al. The role of the microbiome in NAFLD and NASH. EMBO Molecular Medicine. 2019;**11**(2):e9302

[63] Ha S et al. Interplay between gut microbiome, host genetic and epigenetic modifications in MASLD and MASLD-related hepatocellular carcinoma. Gut. 2024;**74**(1):141-152

[64] Liakina V et al. Gut microbiota contribution to hepatocellular carcinoma manifestation in non-alcoholic steatohepatitis. World Journal of Hepatology. 2022;**14**(7):1277

[65] Smith S et al. Reprogramming the Human Gut Microbiome Reduces Dietary Energy Harvest. Frontiers Media S.A; 2023

[66] Allaband C et al. Microbiome 101: Studying, analyzing, and interpreting gut microbiome data for clinicians. Clinical Gastroenterology and Hepatology. 2019;**17**(2):218-230

[67] Mimee M, Citorik RJ, Lu TK. Microbiome therapeutics—Advances and challenges. Advanced Drug Delivery Reviews. 2016;**105**(Pt A):44-54

[68] Vargason AM, Anselmo AC. Clinical translation of microbe-based therapies: Current clinical landscape and preclinical outlook. Bioengineering & Translational Medicine. 2018;**3**(2):124-137

[69] Yim HCH et al. Recent advances in translating gut microbiota research into clinical practice at 12th Asian Pacific topic conference 2023. Journal of Gastroenterology and Hepatology. 2024;**39**(6):979-981

[70] Loomba R et al. Gut microbiome-based metagenomic signature for non-invasive detection of advanced fibrosis in human nonalcoholic fatty liver disease. Cell Metabolism. 2017;**25**(5):1054-1062 e5

[71] Lazarus JV et al. Advancing the global public health agenda for NAFLD: A consensus statement. Nature Reviews. Gastroenterology & Hepatology. 2022;**19**(1):60-78

[72] Albillos A, de Gottardi A, Rescigno M. The gut-liver axis is a key link in MASLD pathogenesis, facilitating microbial metabolite and endotoxin transport in liver disease: Pathophysiological basis for therapy. Journal of Hepatology. 2020;**72**(3):558-577

[73] Hoffmann D et al. Improving regulation of microbiota transplants. Science. 2017;**358**(6369):1390-1391

[74] Verbeke F et al. Faecal microbiota transplantation: A regulatory hurdle? BMC Gastroenterology. 2017;**17**(1):128

[75] O'Toole PW, Marchesi JR, Hill C. Next-generation probiotics: The spectrum from probiotics to live biotherapeutics. Nature Microbiology. 2017;**2**:17057

[76] Aragones G et al. Gut microbiota-derived mediators as potential markers in nonalcoholic fatty liver disease. BioMed Research International. 2019;**2019**:8507583

[77] Bajaj JS et al. Antibiotic-associated disruption of microbiota composition and function in cirrhosis is restored by fecal transplant. Hepatology. 2018;**68**(4):1549-1558

[78] Craven L et al. Allogenic fecal microbiota transplantation in patients with nonalcoholic fatty liver disease improves abnormal small intestinal permeability: A randomized control trial. The American Journal of Gastroenterology. 2020;**115**(7):1055-1065

[79] Xue L et al. Effect of fecal microbiota transplantation on non-alcoholic fatty liver disease: A randomized clinical trial. Frontiers in Cellular and Infection Microbiology. 2022;**12**:759306

Chapter 7

Perspective Chapter: Metabolic Dysfunction-Associated Steatotic Liver Disease as an Emerging Cardiovascular Risk Factor – Pathophysiology, Implications and Clinical Perspectives

Diana-Ruxandra Hădăreanu, Cristina Florescu, Anca Mihu-Marinescu, Veronica Gheorman, Edme-Roxana Mustafa, Adina-Dorina Glodeanu, Rodica Pădureanu, Diana-Maria Trașcă, Ion-Cristian Efrem, Vlad Pădureanu, Sorina Ionelia Stan, Iulian-Alin-Silviu Popescu and Viorel Biciușcă

Abstract

Metabolic dysfunction-associated steatotic liver disease (MASLD) has emerged as the most prevalent chronic liver disease globally and is now recognized as a key cardiometabolic disorder. Beyond hepatic involvement, MASLD is independently associated with increased risks of coronary artery disease, stroke, arrhythmias, and heart failure, even after adjusting for traditional cardiovascular risk factors. Its pathophysiology involves insulin resistance, visceral adiposity, systemic inflammation, and oxidative stress, which collectively contribute to both hepatic fibrosis and cardiovascular disease (CVD). Diagnostic strategies have evolved to include non-invasive tools—such as the Fibrosis-4 Index and Enhanced Liver Fibrosis test, transient elastography, NT-proBNP, coronary artery calcium scoring, and echocardiography—to facilitate early identification of patients at dual hepatic and cardiovascular risk. Complementing these efforts, a novel pathophysiological staging framework for systemic metabolic disorder has been proposed to stratify disease severity and personalize treatment approaches. Management is increasingly multidimensional, combining lifestyle intervention with pharmacologic therapies such as GLP-1 receptor agonists, SGLT2 inhibitors, statins, and novel agents like resmetirom. Given the shared pathophysiological mechanisms between MASLD and CVD, integrated care approaches across hepatology, cardiology, and endocrinology are essential. Recognizing MASLD

IntechOpen

as a systemic disease enables earlier interventions that may prevent both hepatic progression and adverse cardiovascular outcomes.

Keywords: metabolic dysfunction-associated steatotic liver disease, cardiovascular risk, cardiometabolic risk, cardiovascular disease, metabolic syndrome, metabolic disease, multidisciplinary management

1. Introduction

Metabolic dysfunction-associated steatotic liver disease (MASLD), formerly known as non-alcoholic fatty liver disease (NAFLD), has increasingly gained attention as a major contributor to global morbidity. MASLD is characterized by excessive hepatic fat accumulation in individuals with metabolic dysfunction, excluding secondary causes such as alcohol abuse. The shift in nomenclature reflects a more accurate understanding of the disease's association with metabolic syndrome, type 2 diabetes mellitus (T2DM), and obesity. Notably, recent studies underscore the strong connection between MASLD and cardiovascular disease (CVD), making MASLD not just a liver-specific pathology but a systemic disorder with profound cardiovascular implications [1].

Importantly, MASLD is increasingly recognized not only as a hepatic disorder but as a systemic condition with significant cardiovascular implications [2]. Multiple studies have demonstrated a robust association between MASLD and CVD, highlighting its role as an independent cardiometabolic risk factor [3]. This reconceptualization allows for earlier identification of individuals at elevated risk for atherosclerotic cardiovascular events and facilitates a more integrated clinical approach.

The cardiovascular burden associated with MASLD has grown substantially over the past three decades. Data from US national surveys reveal that the prevalence of CVD among individuals with MASLD rose from 8.7% in the 1990s to more than 17% by 2020, emphasizing the urgent need for early cardiometabolic surveillance and targeted interventions [4]. Reflecting this shift in clinical understanding, international guidelines now incorporate MASLD into cardiovascular risk stratification frameworks. The European Association for the Study of the Liver (EASL) recommends routine cardiovascular screening in patients with MASLD and endorses a multidisciplinary approach to address coexisting metabolic disorders [5]. Similarly, the American Heart Association recognizes MASLD as a risk-enhancing factor for atherosclerotic CVD in its latest scientific statement [6]. These evolving guidelines signal a growing consensus on the need to treat MASLD as a systemic disease, with implications for cardiology, endocrinology, and hepatology.

2. Pathophysiological mechanisms linking MASLD and CVD

The pathophysiological interplay between MASLD and CVD is complex and multifactorial (**Figure 1**) [7]. MASLD embodies a systemic metabolic disorder characterized by insulin resistance, inflammation, oxidative stress, and hemodynamic disturbances that collectively foster CVD (**Table 1**). Insulin resistance promotes hepatic de novo lipogenesis while impairing fatty acid oxidation [8]. This metabolic shift leads to hepatic steatosis and a proatherogenic lipid profile—marked by elevated triglycerides, small dense low-density lipoprotein cholesterol particles, and reduced

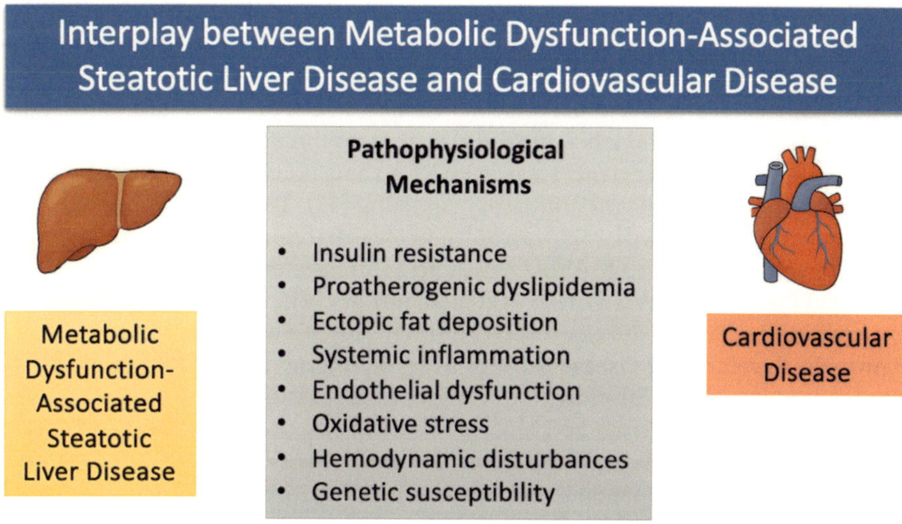

Figure 1.
Interplay between metabolic dysfunction-associated steatotic liver disease and cardiovascular disease.

Mechanism	Description	Clinical relevance	Evidence
Insulin Resistance	Reduces fatty acid oxidation and increases de novo lipogenesis.	Promotes hepatic steatosis and systemic metabolic dysfunction.	Common in >80% of MASLD patients.
Oxidative Stress	Mitochondrial dysfunction and reactive oxygen species production aggravate liver injury.	Triggers inflammation and endothelial damage.	Linked to early atherosclerosis.
Chronic Inflammation	Increased cytokines (IL-6 and TNF-α) activate immune responses.	Drives endothelial dysfunction and plaque instability.	Highly sensitive C-reactive protein levels observed in MASLD.
Endothelial Dysfunction	Impaired nitric oxide signaling and increased endothelin-1/asymmetric dimethylarginine.	Leads to arterial stiffness and hypertension.	Reduced flow-mediated dilation in MASLD.
Genetic Variants	PNPLA3 and TM6SF2 variants modulate lipid metabolism and inflammation.	Influence severity of hepatic and possibly cardiac disease.	Common in certain ethnic populations.

Abbreviations: MASLD, metabolic dysfunction-associated steatotic liver disease.

Table 1.
Summary of key mechanisms linking metabolic dysfunction-associated steatotic liver disease to cardiovascular disease.

high-density lipoprotein cholesterol levels [9]—all of which contribute to atherosclerotic risk [10]. Beyond dyslipidemia, MASLD is a chronic inflammatory state. Elevated levels of pro-inflammatory cytokines such as tumor necrosis factor-alpha and interleukin-6 exacerbate vascular injury and promote endothelial dysfunction. Recent evidence supports a "multi-hit" model in which oxidative stress, lipotoxicity, and adipokine imbalance work synergistically to accelerate subclinical atherosclerosis and impair endothelial homeostasis [11].

Oxidative stress further aggravates endothelial injury by disrupting nitric oxide signaling, leading to reduced vasodilation, arterial stiffness, and enhanced plaque formation [12]. This is compounded by a hypercoagulable state and ectopic fat accumulation in epicardial and perivascular tissues, which promote inflammation, ventricular remodeling, and a heightened risk of arrhythmias [3].

Furthermore, genetic variants such as PNPLA3 and TM6SF2 exacerbate hepatic lipid retention and systemic inflammatory signaling [13]. These alterations are associated with left ventricular hypertrophy, myocardial fibrosis, and coronary artery calcification in patients with MASLD [11]. These interrelated mechanisms underscore how MASLD serves as both a marker and mediator of CVD, and the PNPLA3 genetic polymorphism is a key modulator in this interplay [14]. However, carriers of PNPLA3 variants may develop liver disease without a corresponding increase in cardiovascular events, suggesting a need for more nuanced risk stratification in clinical settings [15]. Other genetic predispositions like TM6SF2 also influence the extent of CVD risk, albeit in variable directions depending on their metabolic expression profiles [16].

Together, these interdependent mechanisms position MASLD not merely as a marker of systemic dysfunction but as a direct contributor to the pathogenesis of CVD.

3. Cardiovascular risk and comorbidities

The association between MASLD and CVD has been consistently demonstrated across diverse populations and is now regarded as one of the most clinically relevant extrahepatic manifestations of this disease [17]. Numerous epidemiological studies have demonstrated that individuals with MASLD are at an elevated risk of both subclinical and overt cardiovascular conditions, including coronary artery disease, cerebrovascular disease, and heart failure, even after adjusting for conventional cardiovascular risk factors, suggesting that MASLD may exert an independent pathogenic role in CVD development [10]. In contrast, another large study examining whether NAFLD independently contributes to cardiovascular risk found that, after adjusting for traditional risk factors, the associations were no longer significant [18]. However, CVD risk assessment remains important in patients with MASLD.

Cardiac structural and functional abnormalities frequently accompany MASLD. These include left ventricular hypertrophy, diastolic dysfunction, and left atrial enlargement—features associated with the development of heart failure with preserved ejection fraction (HFpEF), a phenotype increasingly prevalent in patients with metabolic disorders. Subclinical markers of atherosclerosis, such as coronary artery calcification [19] and increased carotid intima-media thickness (CIMT) [20], are also significantly more prevalent in MASLD. Beyond atherosclerosis and myocardial remodeling, MASLD has also been linked to electrophysiological disturbances. Patients demonstrate higher risks of atrial fibrillation, QTc prolongation, and ventricular arrhythmias [21–23]. The mechanisms underlying these arrhythmogenic risks likely include myocardial fat infiltration, autonomic imbalance, and systemic inflammation. Overall, CVD remains the leading cause of mortality in patients with MASLD, far exceeding liver-related complications, thus necessitating a proactive, integrated cardiovascular risk assessment strategy in clinical practice [10].

Large-scale studies have further validated the association between MASLD and CVD. A meta-analysis involving over 34,000 individuals demonstrated that MASLD confers a 65% increased risk of cardiovascular events, including myocardial infarction and stroke. Particularly concerning is the growing evidence from younger populations, where MASLD is now associated with premature atherosclerosis and increased rates of ischemic stroke and heart failure [24]. These findings were confirmed by a UK Biobank study involving more than 325,000 individuals reporting that MASLD was independently associated with a 35% increased risk of myocardial infarction and a 26% increased risk of stroke [12]. The cardiovascular manifestations in MASLD are often the primary cause of mortality in this population [25]. Additionally, NAFLD is independently associated with valvular heart conditions, particularly aortic valve sclerosis, and mitral annulus calcification. In a population-based analysis from the Study of Health in Pomerania, involving 2212 participants, hepatic steatosis was linked to a 33% increase in the odds of aortic valve sclerosis, even after adjustment for confounding factors [26]. Supporting these findings, a more recent investigation in 180 individuals with T2DM demonstrated that NAFLD posed a threefold increase in the likelihood of developing aortic valve sclerosis [27]. Similarly, a separate study assessing 247 diabetic patients found a significant association between NAFLD and the presence of aortic valve sclerosis or mitral annulus calcification [28].

Moreover, biopsy-confirmed MASLD patients in a Swedish cohort had up to a 2.15-fold increase in CVD risk, while a separate meta-analysis reported a 45% increased risk of major adverse cardiovascular events, rising to 2.54-fold in individuals with advanced fibrosis [29]. Increased liver stiffness (rather than hepatic fat alone) is linked to higher atrial fibrillation prevalence, underscoring the importance of fibrosis as a shared pathophysiological thread between hepatic and cardiac dysfunction [30].

Finally, in a nationwide cohort from Korea, individuals with MASLD had significantly higher incidence of cardiovascular events, including both fatal and non-fatal myocardial infarction and stroke, compared to those without. They also found that MASLD, MASLD with increased alcohol intake, and alcoholic liver disease conferred progressively greater CVD risk, emphasizing the additive effect of alcohol and metabolic dysfunction on cardiovascular burden [31].

Taken together, these findings support the growing recognition of MASLD as an early and independent marker of CVD, highlighting the critical importance of early screening, risk stratification, and intervention.

4. MASLD, obesity and cardiovascular risk

Recognizing MASLD as a cardiovascular risk factor has substantial implications for clinical practice. Risk stratification models now integrate hepatic fibrosis as a prognostic factor, given that advanced fibrosis correlates strongly with cardiovascular outcomes. The CARDIA study revealed that individuals maintaining high cardiovascular health from young adulthood to midlife have significantly lower odds of developing MASLD. Those with decreasing cardiovascular health trajectories were at markedly higher risk for hepatic steatosis by year 25 of follow-up, highlighting the importance of longitudinal cardiovascular monitoring in MASLD prevention [32].

A shared dysmetabolic environment links NAFLD and CVD through mechanisms involving obesity, hypertension, dyslipidemia, and insulin resistance [33].

The natural course of MASLD is significantly influenced by coexisting cardiometabolic conditions. Among these, T2DM is the strongest determinant of fibrosis progression and hepatocellular carcinoma. This dual burden is associated with a 1.5–2-fold increase in the incidence of myocardial infarction and stroke. T2DM also increases the likelihood of developing advanced fibrosis and poses a higher risk of liver-related events and mortality [5]. In a Minnesota cohort, ischemic heart disease accounted for 25% of all deaths among MASLD patients, underscoring the need for proactive, integrated cardiometabolic management [34].

On the other hand, obesity, particularly visceral adiposity, plays a central role in the development and progression of MASLD. Visceral obesity arises as a consequence of impaired expandability and dysfunction of subcutaneous adipose tissue [35]. Visceral fat is highly metabolically active and functions as an endocrine organ, releasing adipokines and pro-inflammatory cytokines that contribute to insulin resistance, hepatic steatosis, and systemic inflammation [11]. Notably, elevated body mass index (BMI) correlates with increased risks of hepatic decompensation, cirrhosis, and hepatocellular carcinoma. Moreover, while a direct causal relationship between MASLD and hypertension has yet to be confirmed, it is postulated that MASLD may promote the development of hypertension through mechanisms involving low-grade chronic inflammation and hepatic insulin resistance [36]. In turn, hypertension and dyslipidemia additively accelerate fibrosis progression. The cumulative impact of multiple metabolic risk factors produces a synergistic escalation in disease severity, underscoring the need for holistic cardiometabolic management [5].

The "portal hypothesis" offers mechanistic insight into the role of visceral fat: free fatty acids and inflammatory mediators are directly delivered via the portal vein to the liver, promoting hepatic insulin resistance and lipogenesis. This may explain why visceral, rather than subcutaneous adiposity is more strongly linked to both MASLD and cardiovascular complications [37].

Adipokine dysregulation is another hallmark of MASLD-related cardiovascular risk. In affected individuals, adiponectin—an insulin-sensitizing and anti-inflammatory adipokine—is typically suppressed, while leptin levels are elevated. Leptin promotes fibrogenesis and atherogenesis, thereby contributing to vascular inflammation and endothelial dysfunction [3].

The pathophysiological effects of obesity in MASLD extend beyond metabolic dysfunction to direct myocardial involvement. Patients often exhibit subclinical myocardial changes, including diastolic dysfunction and atrial remodeling, which predispose them to atrial fibrillation and HFpEF. These manifestations reflect myocardial remodeling driven by chronic inflammation and ectopic fat deposition within cardiac tissue [38].

Obesity phenotypes significantly influence cardiovascular risk. Patients with metabolically unhealthy obesity have increased visceral fat, hepatic steatosis, and insulin resistance, while those with metabolically healthy obesity may still carry elevated cardiovascular risk if visceral adiposity is high. Risk stratification should thus focus on fat distribution and metabolic profile rather than BMI alone [39].

NAFLD has also been correlated with increased epicardial adipose tissue (EAT) thickness. EAT not only shows an independent association with NAFLD, but its volume appears to increase in parallel with the severity of hepatic steatosis, suggesting its potential role in the interplay between liver pathology and cardiovascular risk [40]. Multiple cardiovascular alterations in obesity, including concentric left ventricular remodeling, impaired relaxation, and increased right ventricular afterload, are aggravated by systemic inflammation and neurohormonal activation [41]. Obesity also increases pulmonary vascular resistance and raises pulmonary artery pressures, mechanisms that may culminate in right heart dysfunction and HFpEF [42]. More than 80% of individuals with HFpEF are either overweight or obese, and HFpEF is anticipated to become the predominant phenotype of heart failure in the coming years [43]. Cardiac fibrosis has emerged as a hallmark of obesity-related cardiac dysfunction. Fibrotic remodeling of the myocardium contributes to left ventricular hypertrophy, diastolic dysfunction, and arrhythmias. Elevated levels of pro-fibrotic mediators, including TGF-β and thrombospondin-1, are found in obese individuals, and their expression correlates with the severity of myocardial remodeling [39]. Severe obesity induces profound changes in myocardial metabolism. Increased fatty acid oxidation, decreased glucose oxidation, and mitochondrial inefficiency contribute to impaired cardiac energy production. These metabolic derangements, in turn, promote functional cardiac decline and an increased risk of heart failure [42]. Moreover, studies show that even non-obese individuals with MASLD have comparable, if not higher, cardiovascular risk compared to their obese counterparts [11].

5. Diagnostic assessment

The evolving understanding of MASLD as a systemic condition with cardiovascular implications has prompted a shift toward integrated diagnostic strategies. Current guidelines advocate for a stepwise, risk-based screening strategy to identify patients with MASLD who are at risk for advanced fibrosis and liver-related outcomes [5].

5.1 Hepatic risk assessment

Non-invasive scoring systems such as the Fibrosis-4 (FIB-4) index and NAFLD Fibrosis Score (NFS) are widely used for evaluating hepatic fibrosis in MASLD patients. In addition, advanced imaging modalities such as transient elastography and magnetic resonance elastography allow for precise quantification of liver stiffness and steatosis. In primary care settings, early identification of MASLD using a two-step algorithm—FIB-4 followed by transient elastography—is now recommended. This model has been adopted across several European countries to enhance screening efficiency and timely referral to hepatology. Importantly, the model includes integrated care pathways with lifestyle and pharmacologic intervention aligned with cardiovascular risk profiles [44].

Emerging biomarkers, including cytokeratin-18 and the enhanced liver fibrosis (ELF) score, may further refine cardiovascular risk prediction. These tools provide a holistic view of hepatic and cardiometabolic health, reinforcing the need for integrated care pathways [32]. The latest EASL-EASD-EASO 2024 guidelines support the use of FIB-4 index as a first-line tool, followed by vibration-controlled transient elastography or magnetic resonance elastography for fibrosis staging [5].

Additionally, steatosis prediction indices like the lipid accumulation product (LAP), and fatty liver index (FLI) offer clinicians predictive insight into both hepatic and CVD risk. When combined with imaging, these indices enhance predictive accuracy and can facilitate early identification of MASLD patients requiring cardiometabolic monitoring [45].

5.2 Cardiovascular risk assessment

Accurate cardiovascular evaluation is critical to identify high-risk patients early and guide therapeutic decisions [3]. Clinical assessment begins with detailed history taking for symptoms such as chest pain, dyspnea, syncope, or palpitations, which may indicate underlying ischemic heart disease or arrhythmias. Physical examination should evaluate blood pressure, as well as 24-h blood pressure monitoring,

BMI, and waist circumference to gauge visceral adiposity [5]. Resting electrocardiography can identify left ventricular hypertrophy, arrhythmias, and prior myocardial infarction [46].

Biochemical markers are gaining prominence for cardiovascular risk stratification in MASLD [47]. Several tests are recommended to detect CVD, including high-sensitivity C-reactive protein, serum ferritin, and NT-proBNP [5]. High-sensitivity C-reactive protein is an indicator of low-grade systemic inflammation and correlates with endothelial dysfunction and atherosclerosis [48]. NT-proBNP is a useful indicator of cardiac stress and is independently associated with cardiovascular mortality in the general population [49], and combining it with FIB-4 enhances risk stratification in patients with MASLD [5]. Additional markers such as fasting insulin, apolipoprotein B, and lipoprotein(a) can further refine cardiometabolic profiling [50, 51].

The liver-derived fibrosis scores have also demonstrated utility in predicting cardiovascular outcomes. Elevated scores are independently associated with a greater incidence of major adverse cardiovascular event, including myocardial infarction and ischemic stroke, atrial fibrillation, as well as subtle impairments in myocardial strain [52], suggesting these tools may serve dual roles in both hepatic and cardiovascular risk stratification.

5.3 Non-invasive cardiovascular imaging

Non-invasive imaging plays a central role in evaluating subclinical CVD in MASLD. Transthoracic echocardiography frequently reveals diastolic dysfunction, left ventricular hypertrophy and left atrial dilation in patients with MASLD or metabolic syndrome. These alterations reflect early myocardial remodeling linked to systemic inflammation and ectopic fat accumulation [38].

CIMT is a validated marker of early atherosclerosis and correlates strongly with hepatic steatosis severity. CIMT is elevated in MASLD and metabolic syndrome patients and is associated with increased risk of ischemic stroke and acute coronary events [11]. A 2023 meta-analysis covering over 16,000 cases confirmed a significant association between NAFLD and increased CIMT, supporting CIMT as a surrogate endpoint in cardiovascular risk assessment for this population [53].

Coronary artery calcium (CAC) scoring provides a quantitative measure of coronary atherosclerosis burden. In MASLD patients, elevated CAC scores are independently predictive of myocardial infarction and all-cause mortality. CAC can be integrated into global risk scores for the reclassification of patients with intermediate cardiovascular risk [54]. Finally, coronary computed tomography angiography with pericoronary fat attenuation index (FAI) is a novel imaging modality for detecting vascular inflammation. Elevated FAI values reflect perivascular adipose inflammation and have been associated with higher risks of acute coronary syndrome in MASLD [55, 56].

Collectively, these diagnostic strategies highlight the value of integrated hepatic and cardiovascular screening in MASLD. By combining non-invasive tools with early intervention, clinicians can effectively reduce the dual burden of hepatic and CVD [5].

In addition, in patients with advanced MASLD undergoing liver transplant evaluation, structured cardiac screening using transthoracic echocardiography, followed by dobutamine stress echocardiography, cardiac magnetic resonance stress imaging, or coronary computed tomography angiography is recommended based on the presence of clinical risk factors and findings in baseline tests, with consequent cardiology referral and multidisciplinary discussion (**Table 2**) [5].

Tool/Test	Role	Key findings in MASLD/Obesity
Clinical		
Physical Exam, electrocardiography	Initial risk screening	Identifies arrhythmias, left ventricular hypertrophy, central obesity
Biochemical		
NT-proBNP, High-sensitivity C-reactive protein, Ferritin	Assess cardiac stress and inflammation	Elevated in CVD and MASLD; predicts mortality
FIB-4 index, ELF score, NFS	Liver fibrosis and CV risk	Higher scores linked with major adverse cardiovascular events
Imaging		
Echocardiography	Assess cardiac function	Detects diastolic dysfunction, left ventricular hypertrophy
CIMT	Assess subclinical atherosclerosis	Predicts stroke
CAC score	Quantify coronary plaque	Elevated in MASLD; predicts myocardial infarction
Liver stiffness (elastography)	Fibrosis assessment	Associated with higher CV risk
Coronary computed tomography angiography + FAI	Detect coronary inflammation	High-fat attenuation index predicts acute coronary syndromes in MASLD

Abbreviations: CAC, coronary artery calcium; CIMT, carotid intima-media thickness; CV, cardiovascular; CVD, cardiovascular disease; ELF, enhanced liver fibrosis; FAI, fat attenuation index; FIB-4, Fibrosis-4; MASLD, metabolic dysfunction-associated steatotic liver disease; NFS, non-alcoholic fatty liver disease fibrosis score.

Table 2.
Cardiovascular evaluation in MASLD.

6. Clinical staging of systemic metabolic disorder

Systemic metabolic disorder represents a cluster of interrelated metabolic abnormalities, including insulin resistance, dyslipidemia, and visceral obesity, that progressively damage the liver, heart, and kidneys. Recognizing the complexity and overlapping nature of these dysfunctions, the European Atherosclerosis Society has just proposed a pathophysiology-based clinical staging system to enhance early detection, stratification, and treatment personalization for patients with metabolic diseases. Traditional approaches often treat individual metabolic risk factors in isolation. However, these conditions frequently coexist and contribute synergistically to morbidity and mortality. The three-stage staging system aims to address this gap by offering a structured framework for understanding disease progression and optimizing management strategies across medical disciplines. Stage 1 encompasses early metabolic alterations without overt organ damage. Patients typically present with features such as overweight/obesity, insulin resistance or pre-diabetes, liver steatosis, atherogenic dyslipidemia, or hypertension. Stage 2 involves the onset of organ-specific injury, including T2DM, early chronic kidney disease, subclinical atherosclerosis, metabolic-associated steatohepatitis, or asymptomatic diastolic dysfunction. Finally, stage 3 reflects advanced organ failure or clinical disease, such as HFpEF, advanced kidney disease, cirrhosis, or atherosclerotic CVD. Each stage is identified through the specific clinical and laboratory assessments presented above [57].

7. Therapeutic strategies

The management of MASLD should prioritize both hepatic and cardiovascular risk reduction through a combination of lifestyle modifications and pharmacological interventions. Given the shared pathophysiology between MASLD and CVD, therapies that address both metabolic and hepatic targets are increasingly emphasized in clinical guidelines [5, 58].

Lifestyle interventions remain the cornerstone of MASLD therapy. Caloric restriction, adherence to a Mediterranean diet [59], and engagement in moderate-intensity aerobic physical activity for at least 150 minutes per week are associated with significant improvements in cardiovascular outcomes [60]. Sustained weight loss of ≥10% is particularly effective in reversing hepatic fibrosis and improving cardiometabolic health [5, 10].

Among pharmacologic strategies (**Table 3**), glucagon-like peptide-1 receptor agonists (GLP-1 RAs) have shown substantial promise. These agents promote weight loss and glycemic control while also improving cardiovascular outcomes, offering a dual benefit in MASLD management [61, 62]. Recent consensus guidelines support the use of GLP-1 RAs—including semaglutide and liraglutide—in patients with a BMI ≥27 kg/m^2 and coexisting cardiovascular risk factors such as MASLD [38].

In addition to GLP-1 RAs, sodium-glucose cotransporter-2 (SGLT2) inhibitors remain the cornerstone pharmacological agents due to their beneficial effects on hepatic steatosis, insulin resistance, and cardiovascular outcomes [63].

Statins are another key pharmacologic intervention with proven cardiovascular benefits. Historically underutilized in MASLD due to concerns about hepatotoxicity, accumulating evidence confirms their safety and efficacy in this population. Statins not only reduce cardiovascular mortality but may also offer hepatic benefits, including anti-inflammatory and antifibrotic effects [64].

Drug/Class	Mechanism of action	Hepatic effect	Cardiovascular effect	Approval status
GLP-1 RAs	Incretin mimetic	Reduces steatosis and inflammation	Improves CV outcomes	Approved for diabetes, obesity
SGLT2 inhibitors	Inhibits renal glucose reabsorption	Reduces liver fat and alanine transaminase	Reduces heart failure and atherosclerosis	Approved for diabetes
Statins	Inhibit HMG-CoA reductase	May reduce fibrosis	Strong atherosclerosis benefit	Widely approved
Resmetirom	Thyroid hormone receptor-beta agonist	Improves steatosis	Reduces low-density lipoprotein cholesterol	Approved for Metabolic dysfunction-associated steatohepatitis (F2–F3)
Pioglitazone	PPAR-γ agonist	Improves non-alcoholic steatohepatitis histology	Neutral or beneficial effect	Approved for diabetes

Abbreviations: CV, cardiovascular; GLP-1 RA, glucagon-like peptide-1 receptor agonists; SGLT2, sodium-glucose cotransporter-2.

Table 3.
Pharmacologic treatments for MASLD and their cardiovascular effects.

Furthermore, novel pharmacotherapies are now entering clinical practice. Resmetirom, a thyroid hormone receptor-beta agonist, is the first FDA-approved treatment for metabolic dysfunction-associated steatohepatitis with stage F2–F3 fibrosis. It has demonstrated substantial improvements in hepatic histology and lipid metabolism, representing a major advancement in dual-targeted therapy [65].

Lanifibranor, a pan-PPAR agonist currently under investigation, and pemafibrate, a selective PPAR-alpha modulator, also show promise in improving both hepatic and cardiovascular parameters. These agents represent the evolving pharmacologic landscape aimed at concurrently addressing steatosis, inflammation, fibrosis, and dyslipidemia [66].

Finally, bariatric surgery remains an effective intervention for eligible patients with severe obesity and MASLD. Beyond inducing significant and sustained weight loss, bariatric surgery improves insulin sensitivity, reduces hepatic inflammation and fibrosis, and lowers long-term cardiovascular risk [67].

Recognizing that MASLD exists within a broader spectrum of systemic metabolic dysfunction, recent staging frameworks have emphasized the importance of tailoring therapeutic strategies according to disease severity and organ involvement.

Management strategies differ significantly across the stages of systemic metabolic disorder. In stage 1, the primary focus is on lifestyle modifications aimed at preventing disease progression. As the condition advances to stage 2, interventions must become more aggressive, often incorporating pharmacologic agents such as GLP-1 RAs and SGLT2 inhibitors that address both metabolic dysfunction and emerging organ-specific complications. By stage 3, when clinical disease is established, a multidisciplinary approach is crucial. This typically involves coordinated care among cardiologists, hepatologists, nephrologists, and endocrinologists to manage complex systemic manifestations and mitigate further deterioration [57].

Together, these strategies highlight the growing capacity for MASLD treatment to address both liver-specific pathology and its systemic cardiovascular consequences.

8. Conclusions

MASLD is now firmly recognized as a multisystem disorder with substantial cardiovascular implications. More than a hepatic condition, MASLD is a central component of the metabolic disease spectrum—interacting with obesity, insulin resistance, T2DM, and systemic inflammation to promote CVD. Growing evidence confirms that MASLD independently increases the risk of coronary artery disease, stroke, arrhythmias, and heart failure—even in the absence of traditional risk factors. Given the strong interplay between hepatic and cardiovascular health, diagnostic approaches should combine liver fibrosis staging with cardiovascular risk assessment using tools like FIB-4 index, transient elastography, NT-proBNP, CAC scoring, and echocardiography. This integrated strategy enables earlier detection of high-risk patients and more effective, individualized interventions. Importantly, the recently proposed pathophysiological staging framework for systemic metabolic disorder offers a structured approach to categorize disease severity and guide stage-specific management. By stratifying patients into progressive stages based on metabolic dysfunction and organ involvement, this model facilitates targeted interventions, from lifestyle changes in early stages to pharmacologic and multidisciplinary care in advanced disease. Ultimately, MASLD should be managed as a cardiometabolic disease. Collaborative care across hepatology, cardiology, endocrinology, and primary care is essential to reduce its burden. Early detection and comprehensive intervention remain key to improving long-term cardiovascular outcomes and survival.

Author details

Diana-Ruxandra Hădăreanu[1], Cristina Florescu[1*], Anca Mihu-Marinescu[1], Veronica Gheorman[2], Edme-Roxana Mustafa[1], Adina-Dorina Glodeanu[3], Rodica Pădureanu[4], Diana-Maria Trașcă[4], Ion-Cristian Efrem[5], Vlad Pădureanu[6], Sorina Ionelia Stan[4], Iulian-Alin-Silviu Popescu[4] and Viorel Biciușcă[4]

1 Department of Cardiology, Faculty of Medicine, University of Medicine and Pharmacy of Craiova, Craiova, Romania

2 Department of Medical Semiology, Faculty of Medicine, University of Medicine and Pharmacy of Craiova, Craiova, Romania

3 Department of Internal Medicine, Faculty of Dentistry, University of Medicine and Pharmacy of Craiova, Craiova, Romania

4 Department of Internal Medicine - Pneumology, Faculty of Medicine, University of Medicine and Pharmacy of Craiova, Romania

5 Department of Medical Semiology, Faculty of Dentistry, University of Medicine and Pharmacy of Craiova, Romania

6 Department of Internal Medicine, Faculty of Medicine, University of Medicine and Pharmacy of Craiova, Romania

*Address all correspondence to: cristina.t.florescu@umfcv.ro

References

[1] Rinella ME, Lazarus JV, Ratziu V, Francque SM, Sanyal AJ, Kanwal F, et al. A multisociety Delphi consensus statement on new fatty liver disease nomenclature. Journal of Hepatology. 2023;**79**:1542-1556

[2] Zhou XD, Cai J, Targher G, Byrne CD, Shapiro MD, Sung KC, et al. Metabolic dysfunction-associated fatty liver disease and implications for cardiovascular risk and disease prevention. Cardiovascular Diabetology. 2022;**21**:270

[3] Zheng H, Sechi LA, Navarese EP, Casu G, Vidili G. Metabolic dysfunction-associated steatotic liver disease and cardiovascular risk: A comprehensive review. Cardiovascular Diabetology. 2024;**23**:346

[4] Zhang Y, Zhang X, Huang C, Zhu L. Trends and disparities in cardiovascular disease in US adults with metabolic dysfunction-associated steatotic liver disease. Biomedicine. 2025;**13**(4):956. Available from: https://www.mdpi.com/2227-9059/13/4/956

[5] Tacke F, Horn P, Wong VWS, Ratziu V, Bugianesi E, Francque S, et al. EASL-EASD-EASO clinical practice guidelines on the management of Metabolic Dysfunction-Associated Steatotic Liver Disease (MASLD). Obesity Facts. 2024;**17**(4):374-444

[6] Barton Duell P, Welty FK, Miller M, Hammond G, Ahmad Z, Cohen DE, et al. Nonalcoholic fatty liver disease and cardiovascular risk: A scientific statement from the American heart association. Arteriosclerosis, Thrombosis, and Vascular Biology. 2022;**42**(6):E168-E185

[7] Yanai H, Adachi H, Hakoshima M, Iida S, Katsuyama H. Metabolic-dysfunction-associated steatotic liver disease—Its pathophysiology, association with atherosclerosis and cardiovascular disease, and treatments. International Journal of Molecular Sciences. 2023;**24**:15473

[8] Cusi K. Role of obesity and lipotoxicity in the development of nonalcoholic steatohepatitis: Pathophysiology and clinical implications. Gastroenterology. 2012;**142**(4):711-725.e6. Available from: https://www.sciencedirect.com/science/article/pii/S0016508512001606

[9] DeFilippis AP, Blaha MJ, Martin SS, Reed RM, Jones SR, Nasir K, et al. Nonalcoholic fatty liver disease and serum lipoproteins: The multi-ethnic study of atherosclerosis. Atherosclerosis. 2013;**227**(2):429-436. Available from: https://www.sciencedirect.com/science/article/pii/S0021915013000580

[10] Stahl EP, Dhindsa DS, Lee SK, Sandesara PB, Chalasani NP, Sperling LS. Nonalcoholic fatty liver disease and the heart: JACC state-of-the-art review. Journal of the American College of Cardiology. 2019;**73**:948-963

[11] Ionescu VA, Gheorghe G, Bacalbasa N, Diaconu CC. Metabolic dysfunction-associated steatotic liver disease: Pathogenetic links to cardiovascular risk. Biomolecules. 2025;**15**:163

[12] Targher G, Byrne CD, Tilg H. MASLD: A systemic metabolic disorder with cardiovascular and malignant complications. Gut. 2024;**73**:691-702

[13] Lauridsen BK, Stender S, Kristensen TS, Kofoed KF, Køber L,

Nordestgaard BG, et al. Liver fat content, non-alcoholic fatty liver disease, and ischaemic heart disease: Mendelian randomization and meta-analysis of 279 013 individuals. European Heart Journal. 2018;**39**(5):385-393. DOI: 10.1093/eurheartj/ehx662

[14] Gutiérrez-Cuevas J, Santos A, Armendariz-Borunda J. Pathophysiological molecular mechanisms of obesity: A link between mafld and Nash with cardiovascular diseases. International Journal of Molecular Sciences. 2021;**22**:11629

[15] Santos RD, Valenti L, Romeo S. Does nonalcoholic fatty liver disease cause cardiovascular disease? Current knowledge and gaps. Atherosclerosis. 2019;**282**:110-120

[16] Mellemkjær A, Kjær MB, Haldrup D, Grønbæk H, Thomsen KL. Management of cardiovascular risk in patients with metabolic dysfunction-associated steatotic liver disease. European Journal of Internal Medicine. 2024;**122**:28-34

[17] Adams LA, Anstee QM, Tilg H, Targher G. Non-alcoholic fatty liver disease and its relationship with cardiovascular disease and other extrahepatic diseases. Gut. 2017;**66**(6):1138-1153

[18] Alexander M, Loomis AK, Van Der Lei J, Duarte-Salles T, Prieto-Alhambra D, Ansell D, et al. Non-alcoholic fatty liver disease and risk of incident acute myocardial infarction and stroke: Findings from matched cohort study of 18 million European adults. The BMJ. 2019;**367**:l5367

[19] Park HE, Kwak MS, Kim D, Kim MK, Cha MJ, Choi SY. Nonalcoholic fatty liver disease is associated with coronary artery calcification development: A longitudinal study. Journal of Clinical Endocrinology and Metabolism. 2016;**101**(8):3134-3143

[20] Kang JH, Cho KI, Kim SM, Lee JY, Kim JJ, Goo JJ, et al. Relationship between nonalcoholic fatty liver disease and carotid artery atherosclerosis beyond metabolic disorders in non-diabetic patients. Journal of Cardiovascular Ultrasound. 2012;**20**(3):126-133

[21] Mantovani A. Nonalcoholic fatty liver disease (Nafld) and risk of cardiac arrhythmias: A new aspect of the liver-heart axis. Journal of Clinical and Translational Hepatology. 2017;**5**:134-141

[22] Hung CS, Tseng PH, Tu CH, Chen CC, Liao WC, Lee YC, et al. Nonalcoholic fatty liver disease is associated with QT prolongation in the general population. Journal of the American Heart Association. 2015;**4**(7):e001820

[23] Käräjämäki AJ, Pätsi OP, Savolainen M, Kesäniemi YA, Huikuri H, Ukkola O. Non-alcoholic fatty liver disease as a predictor of atrial fibrillation in middle-aged population (OPERA study). PLoS One. 2015;**10**(11):e0142937

[24] Chung GE, Yu SJ, Yoo JJ, Cho Y, Lee KN, Shin DW, et al. Metabolic dysfunction-associated steatotic liver disease increases cardiovascular disease risk in young adults. Scientific Reports. 2025;**15**(1):5777

[25] Kasper P, Martin A, Lang S, Kütting F, Goeser T, Demir M, et al. NAFLD and cardiovascular diseases: A clinical review. Clinical Research in Cardiology. 2021;**110**:921-937

[26] Markus MRP, Baumeister SE, Stritzke J, Dorr M, Wallaschofski H, Volzke H, et al. Hepatic steatosis is associated with aortic valve sclerosis

in the general population: The study of health in pomerania (SHIP). Arteriosclerosis, Thrombosis, and Vascular Biology. 2013;**33**(7):1690-1695

[27] Bonapace S, Valbusa F, Bertolini L, Pichiri I, Mantovani A, Rossi A, et al. Nonalcoholic fatty liver disease is associated with aortic valve sclerosis in patients with type 2 diabetes mellitus. PLoS One. 2014;**9**(2):e88371

[28] Mantovani A, Pernigo M, Bergamini C, Bonapace S, Lipari P, Valbusa F, et al. Heart valve calcification in patients with type 2 diabetes and nonalcoholic fatty liver disease. Metabolism. 2015;**64**(8):879-887. Available from: https://www.sciencedirect.com/science/article/pii/S0026049515001080

[29] Simon TG, Roelstraete B, Hagström H, Sundström J, Ludvigsson JF. Non-alcoholic fatty liver disease and incident major adverse cardiovascular events: Results from a nationwide histology cohort. Gut. 2022;**71**(9):1867. Available from: http://gut.bmj.com/content/71/9/1867.abstract

[30] Ma G, Xu G, Huang H. Correlation between metabolic dysfunction-associated steatotic liver disease and subclinical coronary atherosclerosis in eastern China. Diabetology and Metabolic Syndrome. 2025;**17**(1):16

[31] Moon JH, Jeong S, Jang H, Koo BK, Kim W. Metabolic dysfunction-associated steatotic liver disease increases the risk of incident cardiovascular disease: A nationwide cohort study. EClinicalMedicine. 2023;**65**:102292

[32] Park SW, Ning H, Carnethon MR, VanWagner LB. Cardiovascular health trajectories and prevalent metabolic dysfunction-associated steatotic liver disease in midlife: The CARDIA study. Journal of the American Heart Association. 2025;**14**(8):1. DOI: 10.1161/JAHA.124.037948

[33] Muzurović E, Peng CCH, Belanger MJ, Sanoudou D, Mikhailidis DP, Mantzoros CS. Nonalcoholic fatty liver disease and cardiovascular disease: A review of shared cardiometabolic risk factors. Hypertension. 2022;**79**:1319-1326

[34] Wakabayashi SI, Tamaki N, Kimura T, Umemura T, Kurosaki M, Izumi N. Natural history of lean and non-lean metabolic dysfunction-associated steatotic liver disease. Journal of Gastroenterology. 2024;**59**(6):494-503. DOI: 10.1007/s00535-024-02093-z

[35] Després JP, Lemieux I. Abdominal obesity and metabolic syndrome. Nature. 2006;**444**(7121):881-887. DOI: 10.1038/nature05488

[36] Zhao YC, Zhao GJ, Chen Z, She ZG, Cai J, Li H. Nonalcoholic fatty liver disease: An emerging driver of hypertension. Hypertension. 2020;**75**:275-284

[37] Lopez-Jimenez F, Almahmeed W, Bays H, Cuevas A, Di Angelantonio E, le Roux CW, et al. Obesity and cardiovascular disease: Mechanistic insights and management strategies. A joint position paper by the world heart federation and world obesity federation. European Journal of Preventive Cardiology. 2022;**29**(17):2218-2237

[38] Koskinas KC, Van Craenenbroeck EM, Antoniades C, Blüher M, Gorter TM, Hanssen H, et al. Obesity and cardiovascular disease: An ESC clinical consensus statement. European Journal of Preventive Cardiology. 2024;**45**(38):4063-4098

[39] Preda A, Carbone F, Tirandi A, Montecucco F, Liberale L. Obesity

phenotypes and cardiovascular risk: From pathophysiology to clinical management. Reviews in Endocrine and Metabolic Disorders. 2023;**24**:901-919

[40] Fracanzani AL, Pisano G, Consonni D, Tiraboschi S, Baragetti A, Bertelli C, et al. Epicardial adipose tissue (EAT) thickness is associated with cardiovascular and liver damage in nonalcoholic fatty liver disease. PLoS One. 2016;**11**(9):e0162473

[41] Borlaug BA, Jensen MD, Kitzman DW, Lam CSP, Obokata M, Rider OJ. Obesity and heart failure with preserved ejection fraction: New insights and pathophysiological targets. Cardiovascular Research. 2022;**118**:3434-3450

[42] Piché ME, Tchernof A, Després JP. Obesity phenotypes, diabetes, and cardiovascular diseases. Circulation Research. 2020;**126**:1477-1500

[43] Borlaug BA, Sharma K, Shah SJ, Ho JE. Heart failure with preserved ejection fraction: JACC scientific statement. Journal of the American College of Cardiology. 2023;**81**:1810-1834

[44] Lionis C, Papadakis S, Anastasaki M, Aligizakis E, Anastasiou F, Francque S, et al. Practice recommendations for the management of MASLD in primary care: Consensus results. Diseases. 2024;**12**(8):180

[45] Laeeq T, Tun KM. Metabolic dysfunction-associated steatotic liver disease and cardiovascular disease. Clinical Liver Disease. 2024;**23**:e0181

[46] Visseren FLJ, MacH F, Smulders YM, Carballo D, Koskinas KC, Bäck M, et al. ESC Guidelines on cardiovascular disease prevention in clinical practice. European Heart Journal. 2021;**42**:3227-3337

[47] Kazi IN, Kuo L, Tsai E. Noninvasive methods for assessing liver fibrosis and steatosis. Gastroenterology & Hepatology. 2024;**20**:21-29

[48] Kirkgöz K. C-reactive protein in atherosclerosis—More than a biomarker, but not just a culprit. Reviews in Cardiovascular Medicine. 2023;**24**:297

[49] Ciardullo S, Cannistraci R, Muraca E, Zerbini F, Perseghin G. Liver fibrosis, NT-ProBNP and mortality in patients with MASLD: A population-based cohort study. Nutrition, Metabolism and Cardiovascular Diseases. 2024;**34**(4):963-971

[50] Ballestri S, Mantovani A, Baldelli E, Lugari S, Maurantonio M, Nascimbeni F, et al. Liver fibrosis biomarkers accurately exclude advanced fibrosis and are associated with higher cardiovascular risk scores in patients with NAFLD or viral chronic liver disease. Diagnostics. 2021;**11**(1):98

[51] Lamarche B, Tchernof A, Mauriège P, Cantin B, Dagenais GR, Lupien PJ, et al. Fasting insulin and Apolipoprotein B levels and low-density lipoprotein particle size as risk factors for ischemic heart disease. JAMA. 1998;**279**(24):1955-1961. DOI: 10.1001/jama.279.24.1955

[52] Lee J, Vali Y, Boursier J, Spijker R, Anstee QM, Bossuyt PM, et al. Prognostic accuracy of FIB-4, NAFLD fibrosis score and APRI for NAFLD-related events: A systematic review. Liver International. 2021;**41**(2):261-270

[53] Khoshbaten M, Maleki SH, Hadad S, Baral A, Rocha AV, Poudel L, et al. Association of nonalcoholic fatty liver disease and carotid media-intima thickness: A systematic review and a meta-analysis. Health Science Reports. 2023;**6**:e1554

[54] Kramer CK, Zinman B, Gross JL, Canani LH, Rodrigues TC, Azevedo MJ, et al. Coronary artery calcium score prediction of all cause mortality and cardiovascular events in people with type 2 diabetes: Systematic review and meta-analysis. BMJ. 2013;**346**:f1654

[55] Yuvaraj J, Lin A, Nerlekar N, Munnur RK, Cameron JD, Dey D, et al. Pericoronary adipose tissue attenuation is associated with high-risk plaque and subsequent acute coronary syndrome in patients with stable coronary artery disease. Cells. 2021;**10**(5):1143

[56] van der Bijl P, Kuneman JH, Bax JJ. Pericoronary adipose tissue attenuation: diagnostic and prognostic implications. European Heart Journal Cardiovascular Imaging. 2022;**23**:E537-E538

[57] Romeo S, Vidal-Puig A, Husain M, Ahima R, Arca M, Bhatt DL, et al. Clinical staging to guide management of metabolic disorders and their sequelae: A European atherosclerosis society consensus statement. European Heart Journal. 2025:1-29. DOI: 10.1093/eurheartj/ehaf314/8125503

[58] Marx N, Federici M, Schütt K, Müller-Wieland D, Ajjan RA, Antunes MJ, et al. 2023 ESC guidelines for the management of cardiovascular disease in patients with diabetes. European Heart Journal. 2023;**44**(39):4043-4140

[59] He K, Li Y, Guo X, Zhong L, Tang S. Food groups and the likelihood of non-alcoholic fatty liver disease: A systematic review and meta-analysis. British Journal of Nutrition. 2020;**124**:1-13

[60] Khurshid S, Al-Alusi MA, Churchill TW, Guseh JS, Ellinor PT. Accelerometer-derived "weekend warrior" physical activity and incident cardiovascular disease. JAMA. 2023;**330**(3):247-252

[61] Alfaris N, Waldrop S, Johnson V, Boaventura B, Kendrick K, Stanford FC. GLP-1 single, dual, and triple receptor agonists for treating type 2 diabetes and obesity: A narrative review. eClinicalMedicine. 2024;**75**:102782

[62] Nevola R, Epifani R, Imbriani S, Tortorella G, Aprea C, Galiero R, et al. GLP-1 receptor agonists in non-alcoholic fatty liver disease: Current evidence and future perspectives. International Journal of Molecular Sciences. 2023;**24**:1703

[63] Genua I, Cusi K. Pharmacological approaches to nonalcoholic fatty liver disease: Current and future therapies. Diabetes Spectrum. 2024;**37**(1):48-58

[64] Bernhard J, Galli L, Speidl WS, Krychtiuk KA. Cardiovascular risk reduction in metabolic dysfunction-associated steatotic liver disease and metabolic dysfunction-associated steatohepatitis. Current Cardiology Reports. 2025;**27**:28

[65] Mousa AM, Mahmoud M, AlShuraiaan GM. Resmetirom: The first disease-specific treatment for MASH. International Journal of Endocrinology. 2025;**2025**:6430023

[66] Lange NF, Graf V, Caussy C, Dufour JF. PPAR-targeted therapies in the treatment of non-alcoholic fatty liver disease in diabetic patients. International Journal of Molecular Sciences. 2022;**23**(8):4305

[67] Sasaki A, Nitta H, Otsuka K, Umemura A, Baba S, Obuchi T, et al. Bariatric surgery and non-alcoholic fatty liver disease: Current and potential future treatments. Frontiers in Endocrinology. 2014;**5**:164